THE CAMP CREEK
TRAIN CRASH OF 1900

THE CAMP CREEK
TRAIN CRASH OF 1900

IN ATLANTA OR IN HELL

JEFFERY C. WELLS

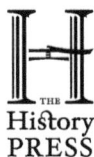

THE
History
PRESS

Published by The History Press
Charleston, SC 29403
www.historypress.net

All images taken by Russell E. Gowin.
Cover illustraton by Marshall Hudson

First published 2009

ISBN 978.1.59629.826.2

Library of Congress CIP data applied for.

Notice: The information in this book is true and complete to the best of our knowledge. It is offered without guarantee on the part of the author or The History Press. The author and The History Press disclaim all liability in connection with the use of this book.

This book is dedicated to J.J. Quinlan, John McDonald, Q.A. Dickson and all of the rescue workers who worked tirelessly to rescue the perishing on June 23, 1900. It is also dedicated to the memory of those victims whose lives were cut short on that rainy summer night. While life moves on, your memories are not forgotten.

CONTENTS

Acknowledgements

T his book is the culmination of not only my work but also that of several people. First, I would like to thank my photographer and friend Russell Gowin. His help in getting all of these photos taken, saved, uploaded and sent to the publisher was invaluable. Secondly, I would like to thank Laura All and the staff of The History Press. Their belief in the validity and importance of my project will never be forgotten. I have read many books released by The History Press, but I never thought that I would be included among the ranks of its authors. Thirdly, I want to thank Susan Prosser, the library associate at Georgia Military College's Atlanta campus where I teach. Her help in tracking down the locations of graves and obituaries helped me find the final resting place of some of the victims of the crash. I also want to thank the reference librarians at the McDonough branch of the Henry County Library. Their help in tracking down copies of the *Henry County Weekly* and viewing it on microfilm was more than appreciated. I would also like to thank Mr. Glen Phillips, director of Georgia Military College's libraries, for graciously allowing me to use our college's databases and historical collection of the *Atlanta Constitution*. My search for newspaper sources essentially started there. I would also like to thank Mrs. Carolyn Beck of the Genealogical Societies of Clayton and Henry Counties. Her knowledge of the history of Henry County and its people is phenomenal. I have oftentimes thought that placing a tape recorder on the table while she talks would be a greater asset than almost any book on Henry County history.

ACKNOWLEDGEMENTS

Perhaps no one I have met loves the history of McDonough and Henry County more than Dan Brooks. From the first day I wandered into Bell, Book and Candle and took the tour until now, he has never disappointed me when it comes to answering questions about the past in Henry County. I also want to thank Dan and Caprice Walker for taking the time to write their book, *Haunted Memories of McDonough*. It was the first book I read from the bookstore. I cannot count how many times I have loaned that book to friends and family from other places to share with them just how "spooky" McDonough really is.

I could never leave out Caprice. I cannot thank her enough for encouraging me. More so than anyone, she seemed to have a fondness for exploring the history of the train wreck. Most appreciated were the many Saturday afternoons when I visited the bookstore and she sat with me as I recounted the many fascinating stories I had learned about the wreck. She always seemed to have an interested look on her face, whether or not she was. I also owe thanks to Shannon, Jan, Don and Melissa. It is so wonderful to meet people who are as interested in the macabre as I am. Keep reading! I also want to thank my colleagues Leverett Butts and Joseph Milford for inspiring me to write. To Dean Roy McClendon and GMC Atlanta campus director Deborah Condon, thank you for taking a chance on a young history teacher years ago and for fostering his love of history and giving him a place to pass it along. Your confidence has always been appreciated.

Finally, I want to thank the readers. It is really for you that I have written this book. I hope that when you read this work, you will understand why I have become such a fan of the history of McDonough and the train crash. To me, these events are not just happenings mentioned as part of the history of McDonough and Henry County. The story of the crash is so much more. The crash is a story of tragedy, heroism and survival. The people I talk about in this book are not just names on a page. They are survivors, victims, lives that were greatly affected by circumstances beyond their control. As I visit the site of the wreck, I can imagine the horrifying scene that must have met J.J. Quinlan's eyes that night as he tried to make his way up that steep embankment. If I could, I would love to sit down with him just once and ask him how he had the strength to make that climb, especially after being onboard the train as it took the plunge into the chasm below. As a teacher, I find the story of Miss Merritt, the Boston schoolteacher from Macon, and her student, Miss Alden, especially interesting.

Yes, to me, the story of the crash is so much more than an interesting tidbit or just one among the many tales of McDonough's past. The trains still run through McDonough, and from my home, I can hear the whistle quite well. Each time I do, I cannot help but wonder whether the sound of the whistle on that fateful night sounded the same.

Introduction

"It was a dark and stormy night." Caprice Walker stood in the middle of the square in downtown McDonough, with the courthouse looming in the background and the statue of Confederate colonel Charles Thornton Zachry in the foreground. People in the crowd smiled, reflecting thoughts that she was about to launch into a fictional account or some undocumented ghost story to heighten their suspense and get them in the mood for the rest of the tour. Onlookers passing by in cars on the streets that wrap around the square glanced in her direction as she prepared to tell the story. The tour historian, Dan Brooks, was standing next to her, wearing his usual camouflage hat. I was one of the participants in that tour, and I must say, as she uttered the story's opening line, I chuckled, thinking about the MetLife commercial with Snoopy sitting at a typewriter. The lines he typed in that commercial were the same as those she repeated. However, the story Caprice was about to tell was not a line from an insurance commercial, and it was no fictional tale. Like all of the stories and historical accounts on the McDonough Haunted History Tour, what the tour group was about to hear was true.

It was the story of the Camp Creek Train Crash of 1900, a tragedy that has been dubbed Georgia's *Titanic*. The crash took place north of the city of McDonough on the Southern Railroad line that connects Macon with Atlanta. The train, carrying fewer than fifty people, crashed into Camp Creek, which flowed under the track north of McDonough on that fateful summer night. Of all the passengers and crew onboard, only ten were spared. The summer rains had swelled the creek and caused the structural

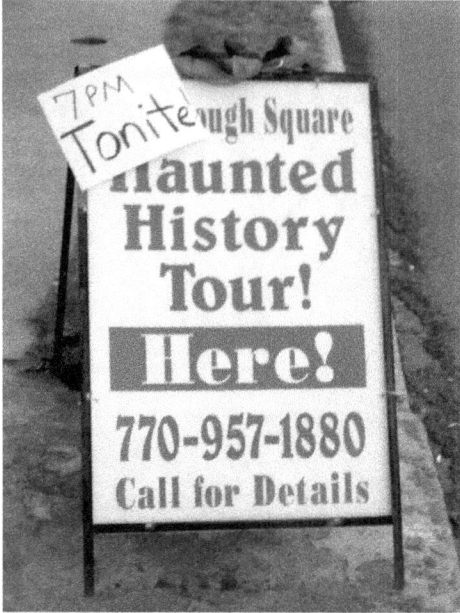

Left: The story of the Camp Creek Train Crash of 1900 is featured prominently on this tour, sponsored by Bell, Book and Candle in downtown McDonough.

Below: Local tour guide Dan Brooks prepares to give a tour of the crash site on June 23, 2009.

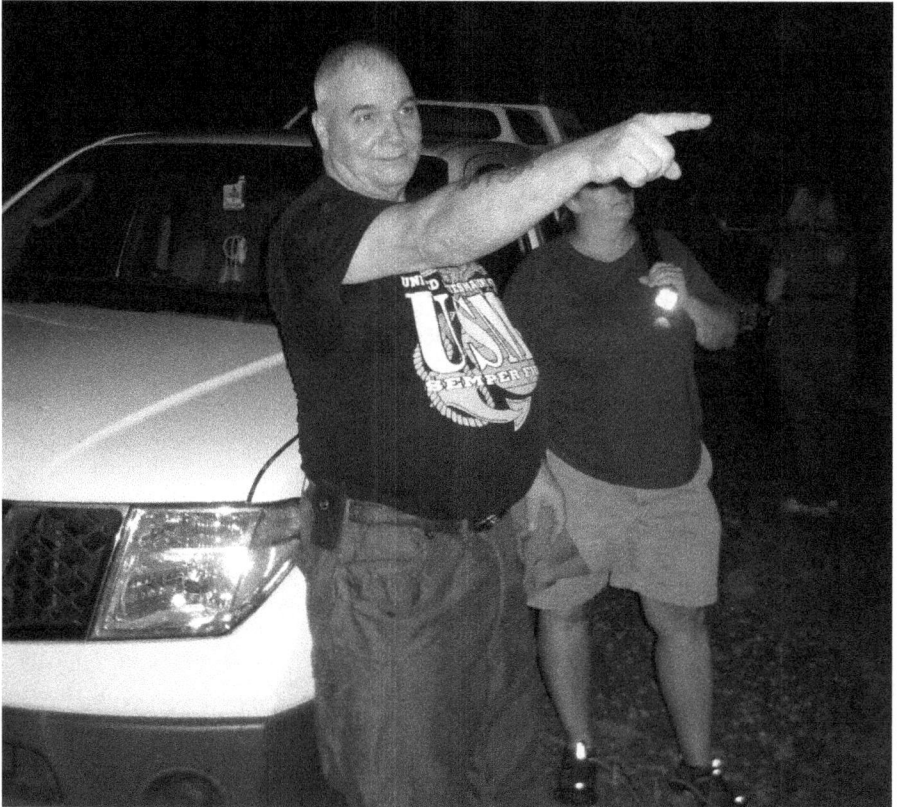

support underneath the track to give way, resulting in the train plummeting some fifty feet below into the raging waters.

Not many people who live in or visit McDonough know about the crash on June 23, 1900. Out on Ivey Edwards Lane, just off to the left, sits the modern bridge above the site. Camp Creek flows gently underneath and is now just barely a stream and not much more than that in a normal rainy season. This was not the case on that fateful night over a century ago. Of course, no one is alive today who was living in McDonough that night. The members of the older generation in the city remember their parents talking about it, but they were not even twinkles in their parents' eyes when the storm clouds released the torrents that knocked out the culvert underneath the bridge and claimed the lives of more than thirty innocent people.

As I sought out more information on the tragedy, I was led to the site of the crash. It was a very moving experience to stand underneath that bridge, right where the passengers and crew of the ill-fated Engine #7 and the cars it pulled plunged to their ultimate demise. I began to dig more and more into the tragedy. I found numerous articles in the archives of the *Atlanta Journal-Constitution*. Our college has the historical collection as one of its many research databases. My next stop was the Washington Memorial Library and its collection of past issues of the *Macon Telegraph*. Considering that the train left from Macon, it was befitting that the paper would cover the crash and its aftermath in great detail. Realizing that the *Henry County Weekly* was only a once-a-week paper, I felt that I would not find much information there. It turns out that there were a few articles on the crash in the local paper, but not as many as there were in the Macon and Atlanta papers. Also invaluable during this search was Vessie Thrasher Rainer's *Henry County, Georgia: The Mother of Counties* and Gene Morris's *True Southerners*. Other informative articles appeared in the *Jackson Argus*.

For information on the history of McDonough and Henry County, I turned again to Mrs. Rainer's book, as well as Mr. Morris's book. In addition, I consulted the histories written and edited by Scip Speer in 1921. Carolyn Beck's short history of Henry County at the *New Georgia Encyclopedia* online also provided a foundation of historical knowledge about the area upon which I built by visiting the Genealogical Society of Clayton and Henry Counties' headquarters at the Brown House in historic downtown McDonough. The society's archives and many files on the history of McDonough and Henry County, as well as family files about the historical figures who helped settle the area, proved invaluable to my research.

As I sifted through all of these sources, I found that, although nothing much had been written about the crash itself, there were a lot of newspaper articles about the tragedy. Some accounts appeared in papers as far away as New Jersey, Colorado and New York City. Also quite useful was C.L. "Buddy" Sealey's article "Camp Creek Wreck Remembered," which appeared in the *Daily Herald* on the 100th anniversary of the crash. Mrs. Rainer and Mr. Morris included small articles about the crash in their respective works as well. While these sources, both primary and secondary, were filled with many little details about the crash, there was no book that put them all together and presented the story of the crash in its historical context. I felt it was important to dig deeper into the events of June 23, 1900, and chronicle the happenings of what was one of the worst train disasters in Georgia at the time.

CHAPTER ONE

McDonough and Henry County Before 1900

H enry County is a thriving part of the Atlanta metropolitan area and sits about thirty miles south of downtown Atlanta. A trip to the area, specifically to its county seat of McDonough, will prove that the area is indeed benefiting from the heavy commerce and expansion brought to Georgia by its capital city. The streets are filled with cars, and the once quiet countryside is now home to ever expanding commercial and residential development. Interstate 75 runs right through Henry County, and several exits on this busy thoroughfare are known as McDonough exits.

As busy and growing as McDonough and Henry County are in the early twenty-first century, there was a time when the area was a vast wilderness on the backwoods of the Georgia frontier. The area had grown a great deal by the time of the train crash in 1900, but one must keep in mind that, at the time of the crash, the area had only been incorporated and settled by Georgians for seventy-nine years. As any student of Georgia history will know, James Oglethorpe and his group of 114 settlers had landed on the coast of Georgia not even a century earlier.

THE COUNTY AND TOWN ARE FOUNDED

Henry County was incorporated on December 21, 1821, by an act of the Georgia legislature and was named for famed American Patriot Patrick Henry. At the point of the passage of the act to incorporate the county, David Adams was Speaker of the Georgia House of Representatives; Matthew Talbot, who had served as governor in 1819, was president of the Georgia Senate; and John Clark was governor of the state.[1] The capital of Georgia was Milledgeville.

At this time in Georgia history, the state was caught in the middle of a long feud between two strong political factions, and Governor Clark was the leader of one of the two groups. The other group was led by George Michael Troup, who was a successor to and protégé of former Governor James Jackson, a political heavyweight in Georgia from 1788 until his death eighteen years later in 1806.[2] John Clark was reelected governor in 1821 by a vote of seventy-four to seventy-two in the state legislature. Clark, who championed himself as the leader of the western farmers and frontiersmen, was an ardent foe of George Troup. Troup was seen not only as a tireless warrior on behalf of state's rights but also as an aristocrat and the icon of the more affluent and established easterners.[3]

Before the settlement of Henry County, the area was part of the Creek Nation. Prior to its incorporation in 1821, the only people who lived here were Creek Indians, as well as trappers and traders scattered about the area.[4] Also occupying the mind of Georgia politicians and their federal counterparts in Washington at the time of incorporation were relations and treaties with the Creek Indians. Perhaps the most significant event in 1821 in this arena was the Treaty of Indian Springs, which was signed between the leaders of the Creek Nation and the federal government. In this treaty, the Creeks ceded all lands between the Flint River to the west and Ocmulgee River to the east. Interestingly enough, the treaty made an exception for the small Creek town of Buzzard-Roost.[5] Out of this agreement came the lands that formed Henry, Dooley, Houston, Monroe and Fayette Counties.[6]

As with every county in Georgia, Henry needed a center of government, which at that time primarily was a place to put the courthouse. That's where the founding of McDonough comes in. The city of McDonough was incorporated on December 17, 1823, by an act of the Georgia legislature. The town was named for Commodore Thomas MacDonough, who was the

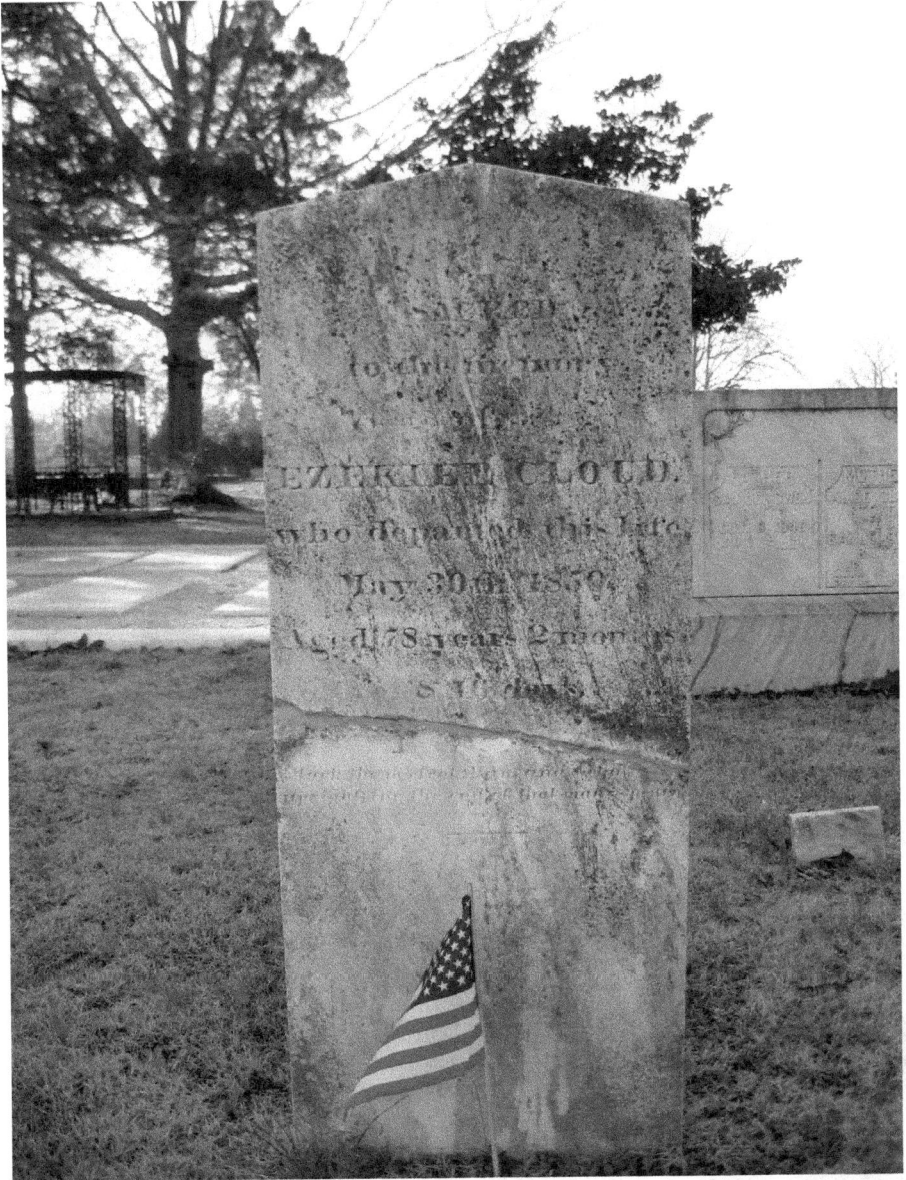

The grave of Ezekiel Cloud, an early settler of McDonough and Henry County, located at McDonough Memorial Cemetery.

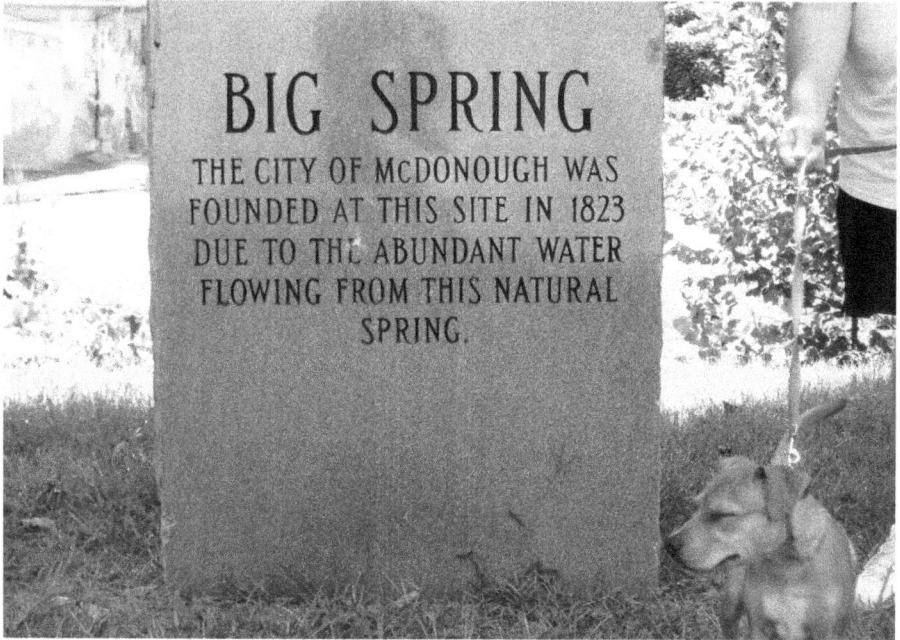

Big Spring, the original site of McDonough. The town actually grew up around what is now the square, just a few blocks from this site.

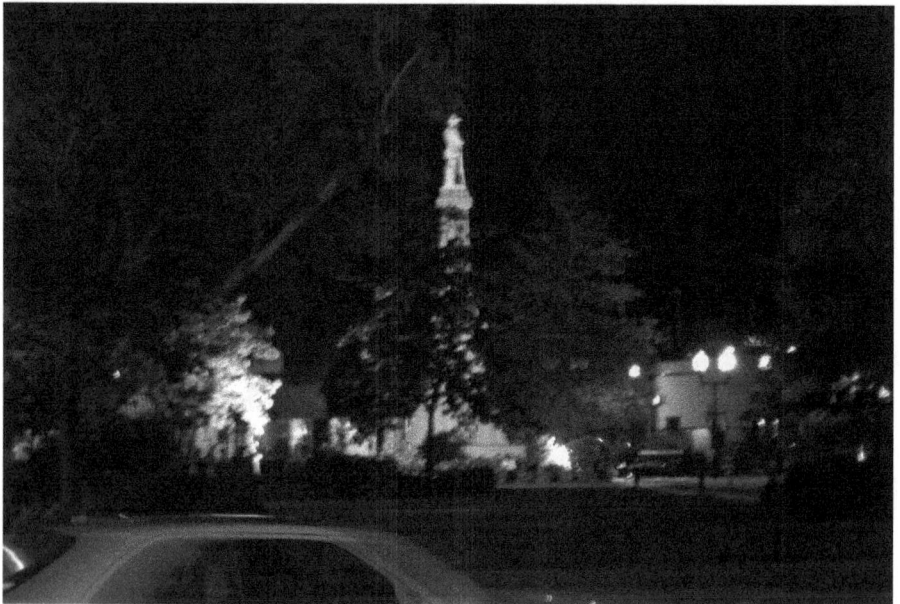

A modern view of the McDonough square. The crash took place just north of this square victor of the Battle of Lake Champlain during the War of 1812. However, McDonough was not the original name chosen for the city that would become the county seat of Henry County. At a meeting held on June 2, 1823, justices of the inferior court met and drove up a stake at the agreed-upon site of the courthouse for Henry County. Those justices were James Henry, William Pate, David Jonson and Jacob Hinton. They declared that the site would be called Henrysville.[7]

THE RAILROADS BYPASS MCDONOUGH

McDonough prospered until the 1840s, when the Monroe Railroad bypassed the city on the western side and the Georgia Railroad bypassed it on the northern side. The cities of Griffin, Hampton, Jonesboro and Marthasville all developed as a result of the Monroe Railroad. Hampton was known as Bear Creek Station at that time, and Marthasville would later be renamed Atlanta. Because the railroads brought so much traffic to these new towns, commerce boomed there. However, those communities, like McDonough, that were isolated from the railroads declined. Merchants and businessmen left McDonough like scalded dogs to go to the cities that were connected by rail. They could not afford to do business in what they thought might be a dying community. According to Gene Morris, official Henry County historian, "Several people even demolished their homes in McDonough and hauled them by wagon to Hampton and Griffin where they were reconstructed."[8]

THE WAR BETWEEN THE STATES COMES TO McDONOUGH AND HENRY COUNTY

As might be expected, the War Between the States affected McDonough and Henry County. It has been estimated by local historians that over one thousand men from Henry County left their homes and went into the service of the Confederacy. However, it may come as a surprise to learn that the delegates Henry County elected to the Secession Convention of 1861 were not in support of Georgia leaving the Union. The three men were F.E. Manson, E.B. Arnold and J.H. Low. These three joined with other conservatives once they reached the capital at Milledgeville and took their seats at the convention. Among the leadership of the conservative wing of the convention were Benjamin Harvey Hill and Alexander Stephens, who would later become vice president of the Confederacy. When the first vote on secession came, Manson, Arnold and Low voted against the resolution. However, they were in the minority, as the resolution passed by a vote of 166 to 130. As the secession leaders, under Robert Toombs and Francis Bartow, drafted an Ordinance of Secession, the conservatives offered an alternative, and again all three of the Henry County delegates voted in favor of the conservatives' alternatives. It failed, and by a vote of 208 to 89, the official Ordinance of Secession passed, with only J.H. Low of the Henry delegation voting in its favor. Nevertheless, all three Henry County delegates signed the official Secession Ordinance as a show of unity with their fellow Georgians.[9] On January 19, 1861, Henry County left the United States of America with the rest of the state of Georgia.

There were several units of Henry County men who went to war between 1861 and 1865, and there were others who were part of the Georgia State Troops and the Home Guard Militia. There are a few whose stories are quite interesting. The first is the most visible in the area even today because he is the man standing atop the monument in the square in downtown McDonough: Charles Thornton Zachry.

Charles T. Zachry settled in Henry County in 1853, having come from Newton County, where he was born in 1828. Sadly, Zachry had the misfortune of losing a wife right as he was going off to war. His first wife, Francis A. Turner, whom he married in 1852, died in the fall of 1861, just months after his unit was organized and left for war. The Zachry Rangers, as they were called, were organized on June 14, 1861. Zachry was elected captain but would go on to rise to the ranks of major and colonel. Interestingly,

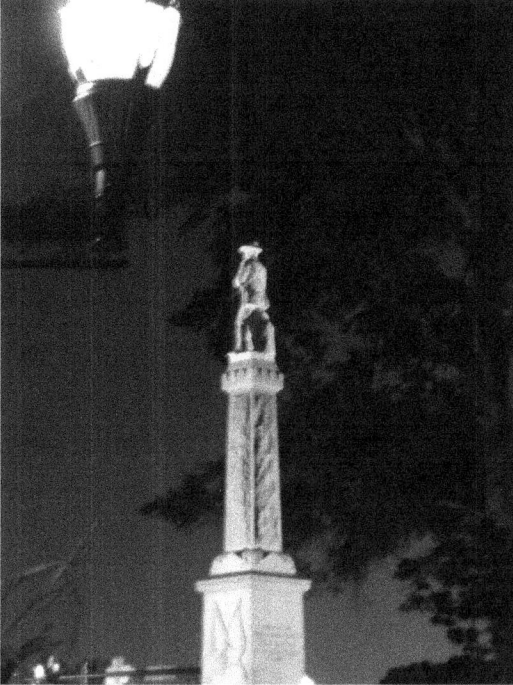

A nighttime view of the monument of Colonel Charles T. Zachry, Civil War hero of McDonough, located in the square downtown.

Colonel Zachry was also promoted to the rank of brigadier general, but the war ended before he could get his commission. In his obituary, it is revealed that Colonel Zachry acted bravely at the Battle of Olustee in Florida; some even credit him with helping the Confederates win that battle when he and his troops made several heroic stands and drove the Yankees from the field. Upon his return home after the war, he was elected as a delegate to the Constitutional Convention of 1865 in Milledgeville, and then in 1880, 1881, 1882 and 1883, the people of Henry County sent him to represent them in the Georgia House of Representatives. In 1890, he was elected to the Georgia Senate. In 1900, Governor Allen D. Candler appointed him judge of Henry County, a position he held until 1905, when he resigned due to poor health. Upon his death in 1906, he was buried at the McDonough Memorial Cemetery in a coffin covered in Confederate gray and draped in a Confederate flag.[10]

The second figure from this era who stands out in Henry County is Dr. Lewis M. Tye. Born in North Carolina in 1821, the year Henry County was incorporated, Lewis Tye came to McDonough as a young man with John Stillwell, who went on to become a leading merchant in McDonough and Griffin. Tye graduated from the Medical College of Georgia in Augusta

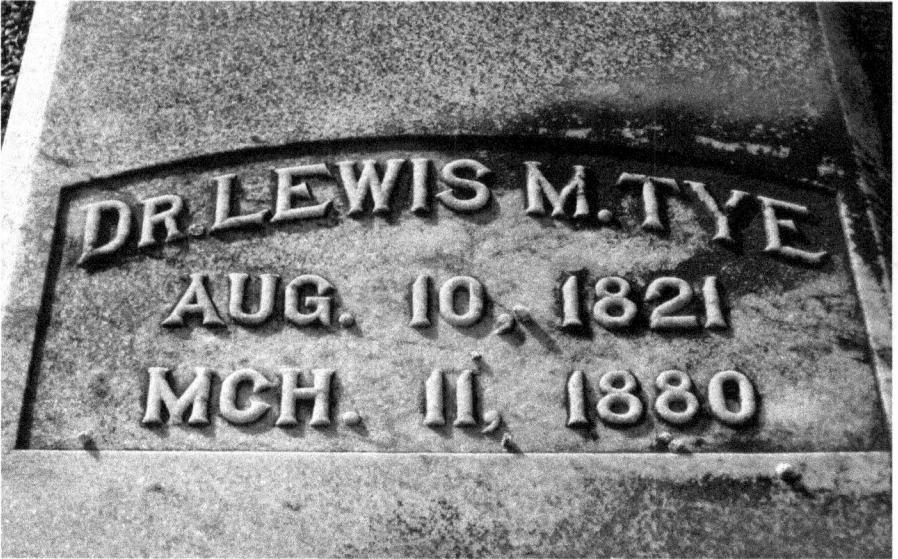

The grave of Lewis M. Tye, a local surgeon who helped save McDonough from being burned when Sherman's right wing came through McDonough on November 16, 1864. Tye treated wounded and sick soldiers in return for the troops not torching the town. He is buried at McDonough Memorial Cemetery.

and returned to McDonough in 1848. Dr. Tye served in the Confederate war effort as a surgeon of the Fourth Regiment of the Georgia State Troops, and many credit him with helping to save McDonough from Sherman's flames during the Civil War when he agreed to help attend to sick and wounded Union soldiers during their passage through the city. McDonough, therefore, did not suffer the same fate as Atlanta, which was partially burned by General Sherman as he made his way through. Dr. Tye represented the county in the state legislature during the war years, from 1861 to 1863. He also served a small stint in the Georgia Senate. For most of the prewar era, Dr. Tye was a Democrat, although most of his friends and neighbors were Whigs. Dr. Tye and his wife, Mary Ann, had eleven children. His son Robert Lee was a physician, and another son, John Lewis, was a presidential elector for Georgia in 1884. He cast his electoral vote for President Grover Cleveland.[11]

Perhaps the largest involvement McDonough had in the War Between the States was as a pass-through destination for Sherman's March to the Sea. Although the city was spared, as mentioned above, the Union troops did stay there for a brief stint.

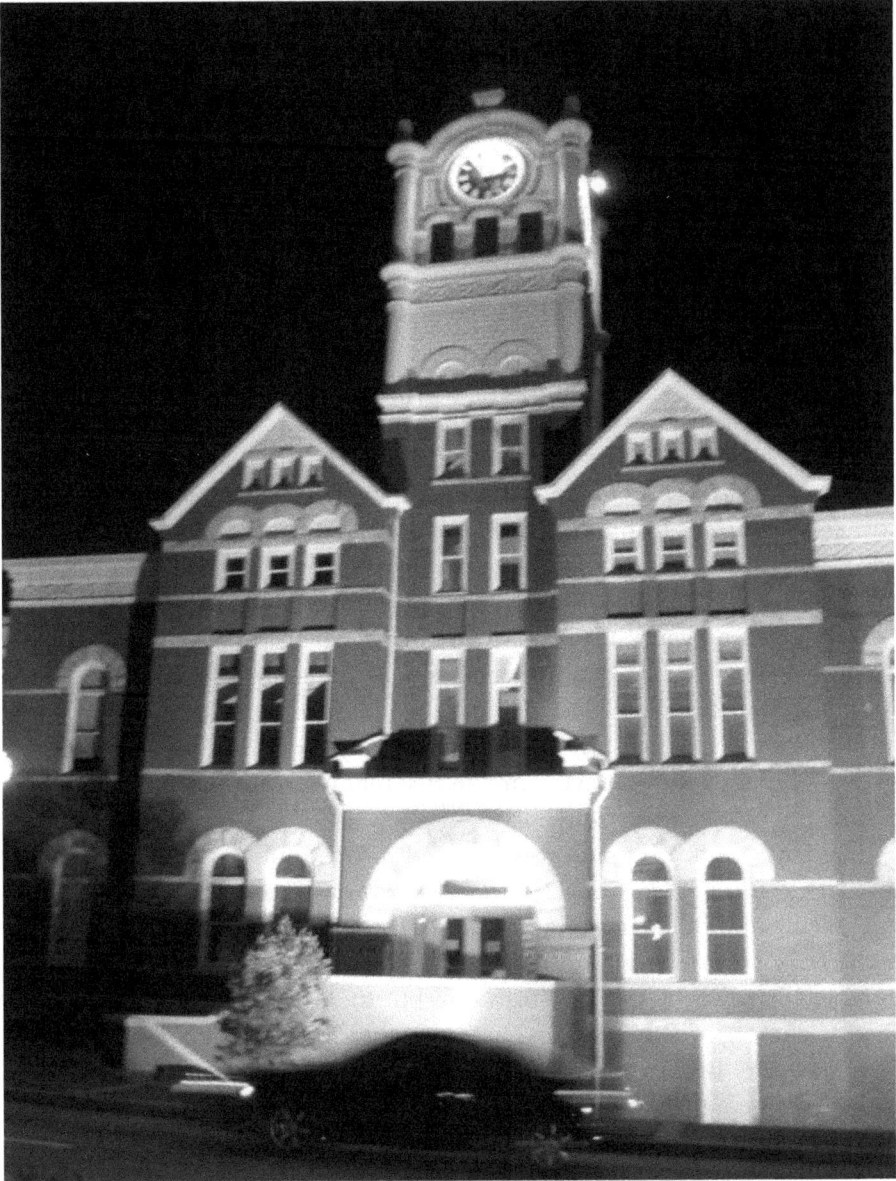

A view of the Henry County Courthouse at night. The courthouse sits on the square in downtown McDonough.

Sherman's March to the Sea began a little over two months after the Atlanta Campaign, on November 15, 1864. The day after the march began, his troops entered McDonough. Contrary to some stories that are told about Sherman's passage through the area, the general himself did not come through. His massive army, which consisted of over sixty-two thousand men, was split into two wings—the right and the left. It was the right wing that made its way through McDonough, and leading the right wing was General O.O. Howard. Included in the right wing were the Fifteenth and Seventeenth Corps. The Fifteenth Corps was under the leadership of Major General P.I. Osterhouse, while the Seventeenth Corps was under Major General Frank P. Blair Jr.[12]

General Howard and the right wing began their march toward McDonough on Wednesday, November 16, 1864. On that morning, the soldiers of the Fifteenth Corps closed in from the west, but they met resistance from the famous Kentucky Orphans Brigade. When the Fifteenth, under Osterhouse, encountered the Kentuckians, they rushed forward, opened fire and sent the Confederate cavalry retreating out of McDonough. At that point, the Fifteenth had a clear path into McDonough. Meanwhile, the Seventeenth was closing in on McDonough after crossing Walnut Creek. Soldiers marched down the Stockbridge-McDonough Road and entered the city around noon on November 16. The city was almost totally deserted, but that did not stop the Federals from arriving in a festive manner, with bands playing and regimental colors flying overhead.

The Forty-eighth Indiana was assigned provost duties, while the men of the Ninety-third Illinois ravaged the town's post office, looking for records, documents and other important mail. All they found were love letters sent home from the war front by Confederate soldiers.[13] Not much damage was done to the town by the Union troops, but there was vandalism at a local Baptist church, which was used as a slaughtering pen for animals. Other churches were broken into, and Bibles, books and other items were taken. The city cemetery, which is now McDonough Memorial Cemetery, also suffered a bit of vandalism.[14]

AT LAST, MCDONOUGH GETS A RAILROAD

After the War Between the States, Henry County and McDonough became very productive in terms of agriculture. Cotton was a particularly successful crop in the county, as well as in the McDonough area. After the War Between the States, cotton production soared, with the average yield for Henry County said to be around twenty-five to thirty thousand bales per year at the turn of the century.[15]

Beginning in the 1880s, railroad construction began to help promote Henry County and McDonough, much as the earlier emphasis on cotton had done. The city of McDonough did not get in on the railroad building in Henry County as early as its neighbor, Bear Creek Station (Hampton). However, one of Henry County's leading citizens, George Whitfield Bryan, took initiative and began lobbying for a rail line through the city. Colonel Bryan was a McDonough attorney and a state senator and was also instrumental in bringing the East Tennessee, Virginia and Georgia

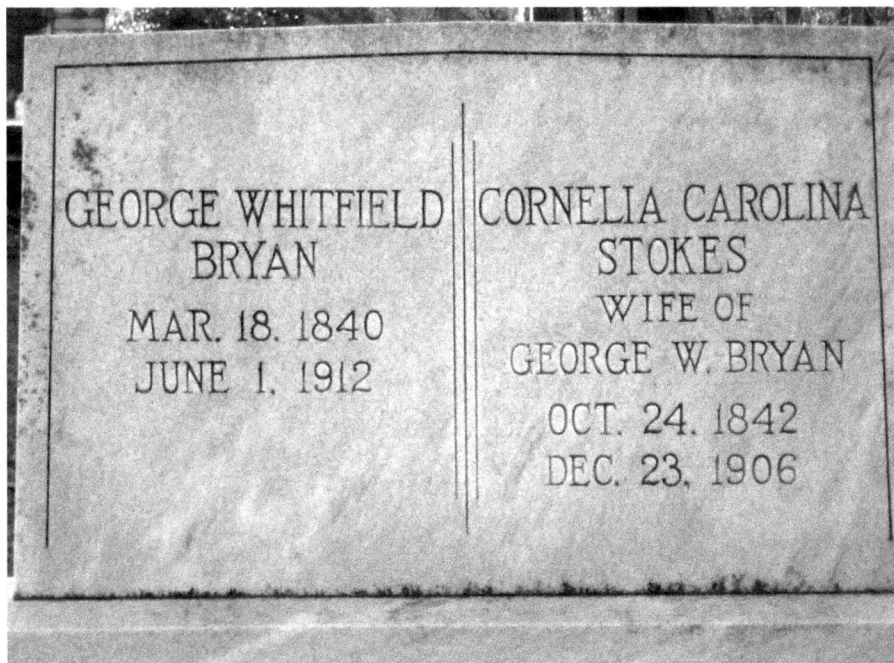

The grave of George Whitfield Bryan, local civic leader and politician who helped bring the railroads through McDonough. He is buried at McDonough Memorial Cemetery.

Railroad through Henry County. He, along with T.C. Nolan, John Nolan and Butts County representative William Smith, lobbied for the extension of the Macon and Brunswick Railroad to come through Henry County. It was announced by the railroad that McDonough would not be included. This decision was reversed on August 1, 1881, and the rail line did indeed come through McDonough beginning in 1882. It was on this railroad line that the ill-fated train met its end on June 23, 1900.

CHAPTER TWO

THE RAILROAD

After the War Between the States, the South began the long trek toward recovery. McDonough and Henry County were no exception. While the area was not overly devastated during the conflict, the economic impact of the war on the area certainly dealt a blow to the local economy. Luckily, Henry County at the time was still a predominantly agricultural region, and cotton production was a saving grace after the war. The building of railroads through the county also helped spur the economy and connected the area with other hubs of commerce and transportation, for example, Macon and Atlanta. The construction of railroad lines had previously bypassed McDonough, but through the efforts of men like George Whitfield Bryan, rail lines made their way through the city in the 1880s.

Mr. Bryan and others lobbied successfully to bring the extension of the Macon and Brunswick line through McDonough. The Macon and Brunswick Railroad was chartered in 1857, but it did not make much progress until after the Civil War. With the influx of outside investment in the railroad, the 174-mile line between Macon and Brunswick was finally completed in 1870. This line was purchased by the East Tennessee, Virginia and Georgia Railroad in 1881.[16]

The East Tennessee, Virginia and Georgia (ETV&G) Railroad was created in 1869 through the consolidation of the East Tennessee and Georgia Railroad with the East Tennessee and Virginia Railroad. When the ETV&G Railroad purchased the Macon and Brunswick Railroad in 1881, it was decided that the new railroad needed an "Atlanta Division." To accomplish this, a 158-mile line connecting Rome to Macon via Atlanta was constructed and completed in 1882. At first, this line was not scheduled to come through McDonough, but through the efforts of Bryan and others, the line did run through the city and started operating in 1882.[17]

In 1886, the ETV&G Railroad was sold under foreclosure, reorganized and renamed the East Tennessee, Virginia and Georgia Railway—not much of a name change at all. It was under the control of the Richmond Terminal Company from 1887 until 1892. However, in 1895, the ETV&G Railway merged with the Richmond and Danville Railroad, and the Southern Railway Company was born. This is the company that owned the rail line through McDonough when Old Engine #7 came through on June 23, 1900.[18]

As the new Southern Railway came into existence, a native Georgian was tapped to be its first president. Samuel Spencer, born in 1847 in Columbus, Georgia, took the helm at Southern Railway in 1894. Raised on his father's plantation, he lost his mother at the age of ten and attended Georgia Military Academy in Marietta, Georgia. He left the academy in 1864 to serve a brief stint in the Confederate cavalry under Generals Nathan Bedford Forest and John Bell Hood. After the war, he enrolled at the University of Georgia but left to go to Charlottesville, Virginia, where he enrolled at the University of Virginia and earned a degree in civil engineering. After graduating college, Spencer became a railroad surveyor and eventually superintendent of the Long Island Railroad. Later, he became the head of the Baltimore and Ohio Railroad. In 1889, he made another career change when he came into the employ of one of the wealthiest men in America, J.P. Morgan. Morgan owned Drexel, Morgan and Company, the firm that acquired the Richmond and Danville Railroad and owned a large stake in the new Southern Railway. Spencer was asked to be the new company's first president. He took office in 1894.[19]

The Southern Railway Company prospered under its first leader. While he was president, Spencer turned the Southern Railway into a prosperous organization. New shops were purchased at Knoxville, Tennessee, and Atlanta, Georgia, and much-needed equipment was acquired for the company. Perhaps the most significant contribution Spencer made to the company was moving it away from its dependence on agriculture, namely cotton and tobacco transportation, to more diversified traffic and a concentration on industrial development.[20] Sadly, Spencer only spent twelve years as the president of the company, a tenure that ended with his untimely death in 1906. In an incident almost as tragic as the Camp Creek crash in 1900, Spencer and several of his guests on a hunting trip were crushed to death by a railroad collision outside Lynchburg, Virginia.

Spencer, General Philip Schuyler, Charles D. Fisher and P.T. Redwood were among the eight people killed in that collision on November 29, 1906. Schuyler, Fisher and Redwood were guests of Spencer as they traveled by rail to his hunting preserve near Friendship, North Carolina, to hunt quail. Spencer and the other men were sleeping in his private car on the Jacksonville Express. Their car, along with five others, was stalled on the track near the station at Lawyers, just ten miles outside Lynchburg. The Jacksonville Express locomotive had gone ahead, not realizing that it had left the cars on the track. There seemed to have been a problem with the coupling as it attached to the mail car on the train. Coming down the track behind the Jacksonville Express was the Washington and Southwestern Vestibule Limited, bound for Atlanta. The Atlanta train, like the Jacksonville Express, was running late and was moving down the track to make up lost time. As the Atlanta train came upon the six cars on the track, one of which was the private sleeping car where Spencer and his party slumbered in this early morning hour, the engineer realized he could not stop.

The Washington and Southwestern Vestibule Limited barreled into the Jacksonville Express. Spencer's car was splintered into what a *New York Times* article called "matchwood." The cars also caught fire, causing burns to survivors and victims. Samuel Spencer's body was said to have been crushed, and it's more than likely that he suffered very little, if at all. He was found under the engine with severe burns to his body. General Schuyler was found underneath as well, but passengers on the train were able to pull his body from the wreckage before his body could be burned. Spencer's private secretary, F.A. Merrill, was thrown from the car as it was cut open and was found lying near the track unconscious. He did survive the wreck. A total of eight people were killed, and ten more were injured.[21]

At the time of the crash at Camp Creek in McDonough, Spencer was president of the Southern Railway. While the trains that ran on the Southern Railway's lines through McDonough were part of a growing, prosperous company that promoted progress and industrialization in the South, the company still accommodated local needs. There was much demand in the area for short trip trains that would run trips of fifty to one hundred miles. The train that crashed at Camp Creek on June 23, 1900, was such a train, making a trip from Macon to Atlanta, a distance shorter than one hundred miles. These short trip trains made many stops to pick up passengers, sometimes at unusual places like side roads and pig trails. Many of the passengers on these short trips were businessmen. The trains also became somewhat of a local attraction, as on almost any given day, young people would make their way to depots to watch the trains pull in and out.[22] Such was the case in McDonough in 1900; however, on that rainy summer night, the weather forced most people inside. Old Engine #7 and the doomed train quietly pulled into the McDonough depot without much fanfare, but its last moments spent trying to leave the area were anything but quiet.

CHAPTER THREE

A Dark and Stormy Night

The rain had set in days before June 23, 1900, and the month had been an unusually wet one in McDonough. In fact, the rainfall for the month had been the highest total in Georgia in over twenty-two years.[23] As is always the case, heavy rains take their toll on roads, rivers, creeks and streams. What is ordinarily a gentle, small-flowing creek at Camp Creek became a small river. The brick support was unable to accommodate the growth of the creek and support the bridge overhead.

For three weeks, rain had fallen on this part of Georgia. Unfortunately, the deluge did not let up in the hours before Old Engine #7 pulled into the McDonough depot. The hardest rain hit the Camp Creek area in McDonough about 7:30 p.m. that evening, just a few hours before the crash and less than a half hour after the train left Macon at 7:10 p.m., headed for Atlanta.[24]

THE ILL-FATED TRAIN PULLS INTO MCDONOUGH AND ANOTHER NEVER ARRIVES

Engine #7 arrived at the depot in McDonough about 8:30 p.m. It pulled a passenger car, baggage car, first-class coach and Pullman sleeper. There were around forty-eight passengers onboard that evening, a number that also included off-duty employees of Southern Railway Company headed back to Atlanta. The exact number of passengers and crew onboard the doomed train is uncertain. The number forty-eight is an estimate based on ticket information and the list of survivors and victims, although those numbers are not exact either. When the train stopped at McDonough that evening, it received orders to await a train coming from Columbus, Georgia.[25]

The train coming from Columbus, #27, is another interesting story in the broader context of the Camp Creek crash. As one reporter for the *Atlanta Constitution* suggested, it was divine intervention that helped prevent dozens more people from dying in the crash. The evening train running from Columbus to Atlanta was to meet the Macon train and couple with it to be taken to Atlanta on the same route. When the crash took place and news of the event began to trickle across the state, there were many details missing, as communication was certainly not as efficient in 1900 as it would be later in the decade. For quite some time, the people of Columbus were left in the dark, as no one was certain if the Columbus train had been part of the crash. One ray of hope did exist. If the crash had occurred south of the McDonough depot, the Columbus train would most definitely not have been part of the crash. If the train crashed north of McDonough, the Columbus train and its passengers most likely went down with the Macon train and its passengers and crew. However, events that night were anything but predictable.[26]

To the south of McDonough is a small community called Luella. The railroad runs right through the area on its way to McDonough. Not spared from the rainfall that caused Camp Creek to swell, Luella and the surrounding area had their own swollen creeks and washouts. In fact, the rains had become so strong near Luella that at Indian Creek the waters had washed out the bridge carrying the Southern Railway lines. Because of the delay, many passengers on the Columbus train were forced to spend the evening at Griffin. Their trip to Atlanta was delayed some eighteen hours. Nevertheless, the delay proved to be a blessing.

The conductor of the Macon train pulled by Engine #7 was William A. Barclay. As the train waited at the McDonough depot, the rain continued. The train from Columbus, part of the Georgia Midline Railroad, was nowhere to be seen. It was routine for the Columbus train to pass through Griffin and then stop in McDonough to exchange passengers before heading to Atlanta.[27] Conductor Barclay did not know that there was a washout at Luella and that the Columbus train would never make it to McDonough.

At 9:45 p.m., William Barclay ordered engineer J.T. Sullivan to proceed to Atlanta, for it was obvious that the Columbus train was not coming. Sullivan signed the register at the McDonough depot, commenting that it was a terrible night and making up lost time would be difficult. However, he also noted that he felt he could get a good start down the long grade outside of McDonough.[28] Survivors reported that the train was moving along at a lively pace. J.T. Sullivan was thought to be one of the best engineers in the business, a fact that comforted the trainmen, even though they were in the midst of a blinding rainstorm.[29] Not everyone on the train felt that way. It is said that

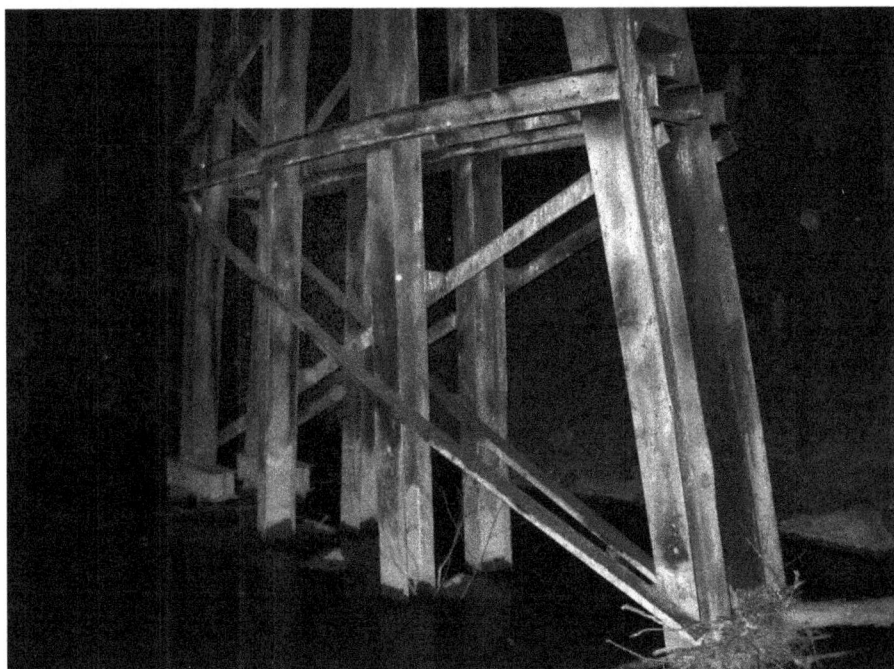

An example of the steel supports that hold up the bridge over Camp Creek today.

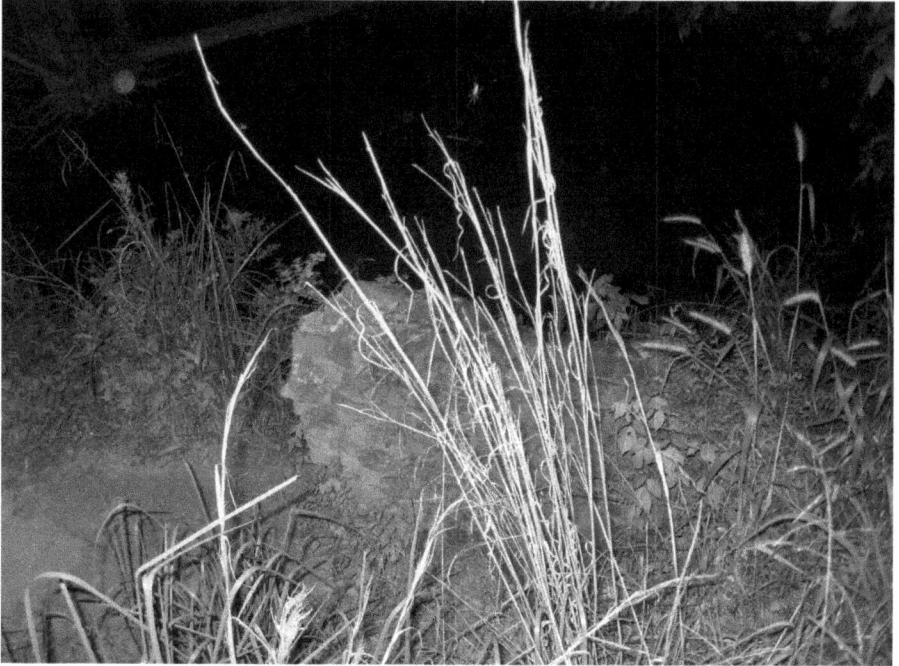

This brick structure was part of the original structure that supported the bridge and was washed out on June 23, 1900. It can still be seen at the crash site today.

some of the passengers expressed concern about leaving McDonough in such a deluge. Alerted by members of the train's crew, Sullivan, following the orders of Barclay to proceed to Atlanta, was said to have remarked, "We'll either be having breakfast in Atlanta or in Hell."[30]

As the train made its way out of McDonough, it traveled along the Southern Railway's line toward Atlanta. The train would have passed through Flippen, Stockbridge, Rex, Ellenwood and Conley before reaching Atlanta, but it wouldn't make it that far. Onward #7 went. On the front of its engine hung an oil lamp to light its path.[31] Fireman Ed Byrd was with Sullivan in the engine room.[32]

Coming out of McDonough, the track curves slightly to the left before it goes down a gradual incline to the high embankment and the culvert that sat over Camp Creek that night. Today, steel supports are in place to hold up the track over Camp Creek; however, on that night, the supports were made of brick, and the strong waters of Camp Creek had weakened those supports and washed some of them away.

CHAPTER FOUR

THE CRASH

M oving north out of McDonough, Sullivan set his levers and allowed the train to progress. Onboard was passenger E.S. Schriever. He was in the passenger (Pullman) car and was able to recount the events leading up to the crash. According to Schriever, there were four people in the smoking compartment of the sleeping car. Besides Schriever, there were Mr. E.T. Mack of Chattanooga, Walter Pope of Atlanta and J.C. Flynn of Flovilla, all of whom survived the crash. Although he was unsure of how quickly the train was moving, Schriever remarked that it seemed to be going along quite rapidly. He saw and heard the rain pouring down furiously but did mention that everyone in the sleeper seemed quite comfortable. Two ladies who also survived the crash—a Miss Merritt, who was a schoolteacher in Boston, and her student, Miss Clara Alden—were in the center of the sleeping car. The two had been visiting Macon. Schriever could hear Alden and Merritt talking a short distance away from him.

The porter, T.C. Carter, also a survivor, left the smoking compartment shortly before the crash and had moved toward Miss Alden and Miss Merritt to attend to them. In his account, Schriever mentioned that the conductor, H.R. Cressman of Asheville, North Carolina, who unfortunately did not survive, was in the forward end of the sleeping car at the time. Suddenly, he reported, and without any warning, there was a jerk as if the engineer had applied the emergency brakes. The next thing he remembered was crashing. To his recollection, everything went dark and water came rushing into the car. No sounds could be heard from the other cars.[33]

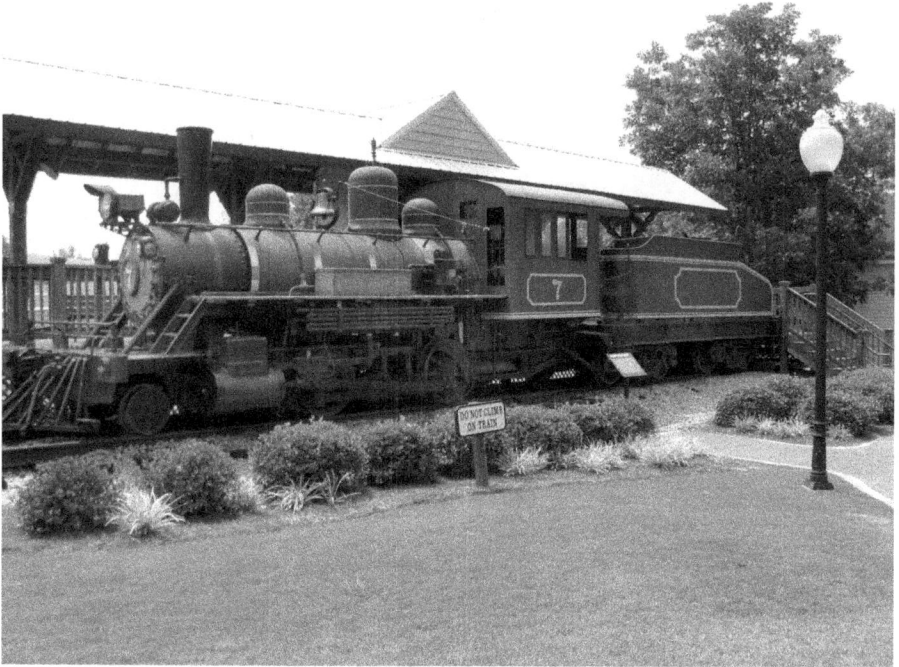

In Heritage Park in McDonough sits this replica of Old # 7, the engine that drove the train that crashed in Camp Creek on June 23, 1900.

When the car stopped rolling, those who could began to climb out, according to Schriever. The Pullman car rested with one end on the abutment of a trestle, or possibly a culvert. The back end seemed to rest on the embankment. Schriever also mentioned that the car was broken in the center, and there were exposed pipes all over the place, as well as much debris.[34] Pictures submitted to various newspapers after the wreck show the Pullman car resting in the position that Schriever described.

Schriever mentioned that he and four others climbed out of the Pullman car and reached the embankment. They climbed to the roof of the car and stayed there for two hours, enduring the pounding rain. J.C. Flynn attempted to climb up the embankment, but he struggled and fell back into the water. The stream, strong and swift, swept him down the creek almost a half mile. Perhaps saving his life, he caught himself on a stump and finally reached the bank. He was quite exhausted and almost devoid of life; however, he was lucky enough to be counted among the survivors.[35] The other survivor who attempted to climb the embankment was the train's flagman, J.J. Quinlan.

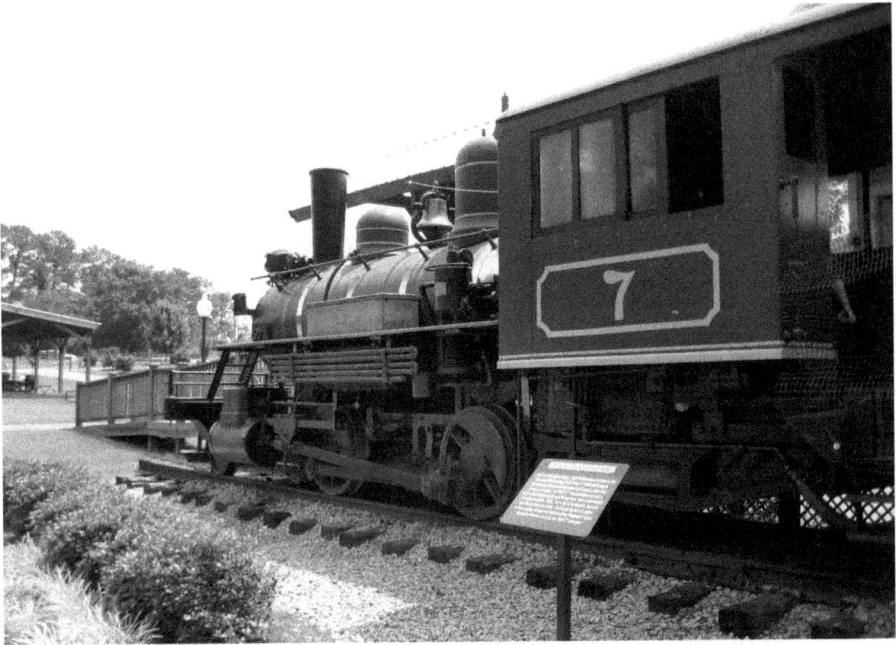

Another view of the replica of Old #7 in Heritage Park, not far from the crash site.

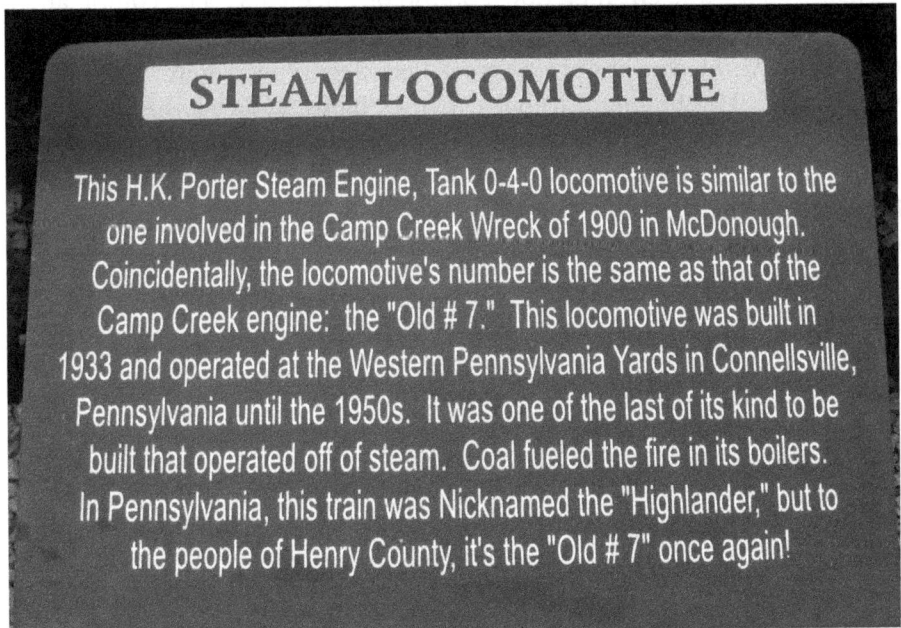

STEAM LOCOMOTIVE

This H.K. Porter Steam Engine, Tank 0-4-0 locomotive is similar to the one involved in the Camp Creek Wreck of 1900 in McDonough. Coincidentally, the locomotive's number is the same as that of the Camp Creek engine: the "Old # 7." This locomotive was built in 1933 and operated at the Western Pennsylvania Yards in Connellsville, Pennsylvania until the 1950s. It was one of the last of its kind to be built that operated off of steam. Coal fueled the fire in its boilers. In Pennsylvania, this train was Nicknamed the "Highlander," but to the people of Henry County, it's the "Old # 7" once again!

The plaque that explains the replica of Old # 7.

As he climbed, he loosened dirt and crossties. However, he did manage to reach the tracks above. He yelled to the surviving passengers and crew that he was going to head back to McDonough to flag a train headed this way and get some help.

Schriever reported that others tried to climb the embankment, but because of wet sand and mud, none were successful. At some point, a man came to the edge of the bank above the survivors, and the group asked him to throw down a rope to pull them up. After some time spent looking for rope, the rescuer threw down a line and pulled up survivors, dragging them through mud and sand. Everyone who was alive in the sleeper was pulled up this way, and they walked back to McDonough. There they remained for a few days. Some of them were taken to Hampton to catch a northbound train. Schriever reported that once he was pulled to safety and began his walk back to McDonough, he never returned to the crash site. In his words, he "had no desire to see the terrible sight [he] witnessed at intervals through the night by the glare of the burning coaches and the flashes of lighting."[36]

Indeed, the sight was a terrible one. When Sullivan approached the bridge, he threw on the brakes to try to bring the train to a halt, but with no success. The washout at the bridge was roughly the size of about two car lengths. The regular coach came crashing down on top of the engine. The combination coach and the sleeper coach swung around and landed downstream of the other cars. As the coaches hit the creek bed, they immediately began filling with water.[37] The Pullman sleeper car stuck halfway out of the water, and more than anything, this is what saved the passengers onboard. The only victim from the Pullman was Conductor Cressman. It was later reported by survivors that they remembered him being at the front end of the coach reading a book as the train crashed.[38]

CHAPTER FIVE

THE HEROES

T ragedy generally opens the doors for heroism, and the Camp Creek crash was no different. While there is sometimes a dearth of information on what happened at any given point, there was certainly no shortage of heroes. While it is difficult to judge acts of heroism and kindness and signal one as greater than the next, the acts of Southern Railway flagman J.J. Quinlan certainly stand out.

J.J. QUINLAN SAVES MORE LIVES

As one of only ten survivors, as well as an employee of the railroad, it was quite natural for reporters and interested parties to want to speak with Quinlan. He lived in Macon at the time of the crash, and the *Macon Telegraph* reported that he had come to Macon as a youth, with no money and no friends. Apparently, at some point shortly after he came to Macon, he was arrested for vagrancy, something that commonly happened to newcomers to an area who had nothing and made their way to the cities for work. A local lady by the name of Mrs. McKenna eventually took pity on the young boy and offered him a job in her store on Fourth Street. Trustworthy and smart, Quinlan earned friends quickly. Over time, he worked hard and was eventually offered a position with the Macon and Indian Springs Railroad, where he worked as a conductor. Eventually, he worked for the Consolidated Railroad as a streetcar man. At the time of the crash at Camp Creek, he had been with the Southern Railway for only a few months.[39]

Interviews with Quinlan were carried in almost all of the major papers in Georgia offering news of the tragedy. In his testimony, Quinlan recalled that when the train left McDonough, he was seated in the front end of the sleeper car. He mentioned that the crash came so quickly that he had hardly had enough time to get settled. He said that there were two ladies in the sleeper car with him. (Based on other testimony, these ladies were Miss Merritt and Miss Alden.) This makes it clear that he was in the Pullman car at the end of the train. He also mentioned that there were some men seated near him. Everyone appeared comfortable, he thought, as the train made its way toward its Atlanta destination. Then, without warning, he felt the air brakes applied, noting that they had been turned on with a jerk.[40] Quinlan's account, along with those of Schriever and others, mentions that Sullivan applied the brakes as he approached the Camp Creek Bridge. There has been some debate about this. As pictures of the wreck illustrate, the engine was on the other side of the chasm, which has led to speculation that Sullivan may have tried to speed up in hopes of making it to the other side. However, the testimonies of more than one survivor, one of whom was a trained railroad employee, give credence to the notion that Sullivan did apply the brakes in an attempt to stop the train before it came to the bridge.

When Quinlan felt the brakes being applied, he realized that something was wrong, but he had no time to act because the train crashed only seconds later. At that point, he found himself being thrown about and then jammed into the corner of the sleeper car. One of the berths fell on top of him. Glass fell in around him, and water started to rush into the car. He recounted that he "fought to get loose from [his] penning, but could not see a thing. It was as dark and silent as the grave."[41]

Thinking that he might be trapped, he looked around in all directions. At first he heard the sound of what he thought was crashing timbers but deduced that it was the sound of the train cars falling on top of one another. Afterward, no sounds could be heard, and for a few moments Quinlan thought he might be the only person alive on the train. It was dark, and as he continued to look around, he could see nothing. Then he noticed some light filtering through in one direction. He decided to move as best he could toward that light. Reaching that area, he discovered that it was the end of the sleeper sticking out of the water.[42] From this account, it appears that at first Quinlan was trapped in the end of the sleeper car that was underneath the water, and he could easily have been one of the victims. He was quite lucky to have made it out alive.

As mentioned earlier, Miss Mamie Merritt, the Boston schoolteacher, was on that sleeper with Quinlan. She remembered that when the train left Macon, the rain was already coming down pretty hard. The rain continued all the way to McDonough, according to her testimony. A conductor, one she did not name, came to her seat and asked her if he could let down her window since the rain was coming in so forcefully. She consented and then reached to gather the sewing materials spread out on her lap. The train had only been moving north of McDonough at that point for five minutes or so. It was when she bent forward to gather her sewing that the crash occurred. Looking up with a start, she saw the conductor who had helped her with her window being thrown headlong to the front of the sleeper car. She was seated on the left of the car, and Miss Alden was seated on the right. She remembered the car plunging downward. The car turned over onto its left side. The impact caused Miss Alden to be thrown over the seats on top of Miss Merritt, and Miss Merritt could hear the girl crying loudly. The water was rising quickly, and before they knew it, it had risen to their waists. Seeing that Miss Alden's head was dangerously near the water, Miss Merritt took her in her arms and lifted her. They were both wedged in and could not move anything below their waists. They lay there for a few moments, helpless. The only thing they could do was cry for help.[43]

When no one answered their cries for help, Miss Merritt realized that she and Miss Alden were going to have to help themselves. Miss Alden was trapped by a steam pipe across her body. Taking a wooden beam, Miss Merritt kept working and finally dislodged the steam pipe, freeing Miss Alden. Miss Merritt, however, was partially trapped by a partition that had fallen on her. She began working her way out from underneath its grip and managed to free herself. She then crawled over to the broken part of the sleeper car and looked out through the opening. By this time, Quinlan and Flynn had emerged on top of the sleeper and were trying to climb the embankment. She called to them, but they could not hear her. However, Porter T.C. Carter, an African American who worked on the Pullman car, did hear her cries. He came to help, but his dislocated hip prevented him from doing much good.[44]

When Quinlan finally made his way to the top of the Pullman sleeper, he said it was quite dark and he could hardly make out which way was which. He was holding an oil lantern, which he discerned was the only light still burning at the time. From his statements, one can assume that the coaches and engine had yet to catch fire. Standing there, he felt that he needed to try to make his way back to McDonough to stop the freight train that was on its way down the same stretch of track. While some might argue that Quinlan should have worked to rescue passengers and crew, his decision to wave down an oncoming train was the right one, for if that train had not been waved off, it would have plunged into Camp Creek as well, killing everyone onboard that train and possibly killing any survivors of the first wreck.

While Quinlan was on top of the sleeper attempting to find a way to the tracks above, another person appeared through the opening of the back end of the sleeper—J.C. Flynn. Quinlan mentions that Flynn asked him for his lantern, but he told Flynn that it was too dangerous and that the sleeper car was in serious jeopardy. Flynn decided to climb onboard the sleeper with Quinlan. There, Flynn convinced Quinlan to allow him to hold his lantern while he (Quinlan) climbed the embankment to the tracks overhead. Quinlan remarked that the embankment appeared to be—and, as he learned when he started to climb, was—as steep as a pine tree. Nevertheless, the two men knew that one of them had to make it to the tracks and back to McDonough to warn the oncoming train and to alert the town of what had happened so they could round up as much help as possible for the rescue of survivors.[45]

T.C. Carter was determined to get help for Miss Merritt and Miss Alden. He crawled to the opening of the sleeper car and yelled for help from Quinlan and Flynn. They were unable to respond, so Carter returned to the ladies. With his help, Miss Merritt was able to help Miss Alden to the roof of the sleeper, where someone could rescue her more easily. In her comments, Miss Merritt credited T.C. Carter with helping the two ladies survive the crash. It must be kept in mind that his acts were accomplished as he struggled against the pain of a dislocated hip. The ladies themselves suffered a fair amount of injuries. Miss Merritt had a bad cut on her hand, a cut on her left cheek and a deep cut on her left arm. Miss Alden suffered a severe cut on her right arm and was badly bruised all over, much like her friend.[46]

The Heroes

It was while the ladies were struggling to get to the top of the sleeper car that Quinlan began climbing his way up the embankment, all the while fighting the loose dirt and steepness of the climb. As he struggled, he fell back down, dragging dirt with him. The task became quite arduous, and the depth of Quinlan's heroism became apparent in the face of the difficulties he eventually overcame. Over and over he tried and failed. At one point, he felt that he would have to give up and lie wherever he landed due to exhaustion. Thoughts of the oncoming freight train ran through his head, but he doubted he could go on. It was at this time that a few people yelled out to him from the sleeper car to not give up and try again. He got up again and kept trying. At one point, he looked behind him to survey the scene in case there was a better route to the top than the one he was trying to take. He noticed that the first-class coach and the baggage car had caught fire. Thinking it odd that the cars would catch fire while submerged in the waters of Camp Creek, he realized that they were going to be engulfed quickly. He also thought about the people who were in those cars and how he hoped, and was almost certain, that they had been killed instantly. If there was a comforting thought associated with this hellish scene, it was that these people did not suffer. Realizing that the scene would become even more of a nightmare if the oncoming freight train was allowed to come through unwarned, Quinlan was determined to keep moving and make it to McDonough.[47]

The situation was growing more and more intense with each passing moment. Quinlan recalled that he "dug [his] fingers deep into the mud and squeezed the ground as hard as [he] could with [his] knees." Determined not to give up, he lunged forward and finally felt his hand gripping a crosstie, a sign that he had reached the top of the embankment and was near the track. This was confirmed when he heard the voices of those on the sleeper car cheering his accomplishment. The moment of exhilaration was temporary, for seconds later, those cheering voices were drowned out by the sounds of the collapsing embankment below him. It was quite fortunate that he made it to the top when he did; otherwise, he would have crashed into the creek. In fact, Quinlan reported that the man with his lantern, whom we now know was Flynn, fell headfirst into the creek and was swept downstream, only to be found a mile and a half down creek holding tightly to a stump. Quinlan said that he saw Flynn about an hour later when he was taken to McDonough with other men from the wreck.[48]

Now on the track, Quinlan knew that he had to make a quick dash for the McDonough depot so that railroad officials there could call off the freight train's run to Atlanta. As he made his way up the track, he passed the houses of several African American families. Waking them up, he told them of the wreck and said that their help was needed to rescue survivors. He instructed them to gather all of the rope they could find and take it with them to the washout. Quinlan knew that this was the only way the survivors could be pulled out of the chasm below the tracks. Although unnamed, these African American residents near McDonough responded quickly and heroically.[49]

From later testimony, we know that the African Americans who lived near the track must have alerted others living in the area. One of the men alerted was John A. McDonald. McDonald testified that he was awakened by an African American (no gender is given) and informed of the crash. McDonald was one of the first people to arrive on the scene, although it is quite possible that Q.A. Dickson was there before him. Upon surveying the damage, McDonald took off a good bit of his clothing so that he could work more freely in the water below. One of the first things he noticed was a man bobbing up and down in the creek and then being swept away. McDonald mentioned that the groaning and screams coming from the scene were tormenting. He could see a man moving about on a burning car. Realizing that the man was in for a hellish nightmare once the flames engulfing the car reached his end of the compartment, McDonald swore to make his best attempt to rescue the man. A good swimmer, McDonald quickly made his way to the car. The man he was trying to save was Conductor J.E. Woods. He made his way to Woods and pulled him from the burning sleeper car. Dragging him into the water, McDonald fought the current and carried Woods to the creek bank. When the two reached the bank, Woods spoke to his rescuer. His words were: "Tell Jim—tell Jim—railroad—" Woods never finished that sentence. McDonald had behaved heroically in trying to save Woods, but the extent of his injuries were greater than the feat of bravery, and Camp Creek claimed another victim.[50]

Quinlan finally reached the McDonough depot. In what could only be called divine intervention, just as he arrived, the northbound freight train pulled into the depot. One must pause and consider the depth of this situation. If Quinlan had stopped along the track to McDonough to rest, as he most certainly was entitled to do after his feat of climbing that steep embankment at the creek, the train may have easily left the depot and not been able to stop before coming on the washed-out bridge at Camp Creek. Or perhaps if Quinlan had stopped trying to climb the embankment until

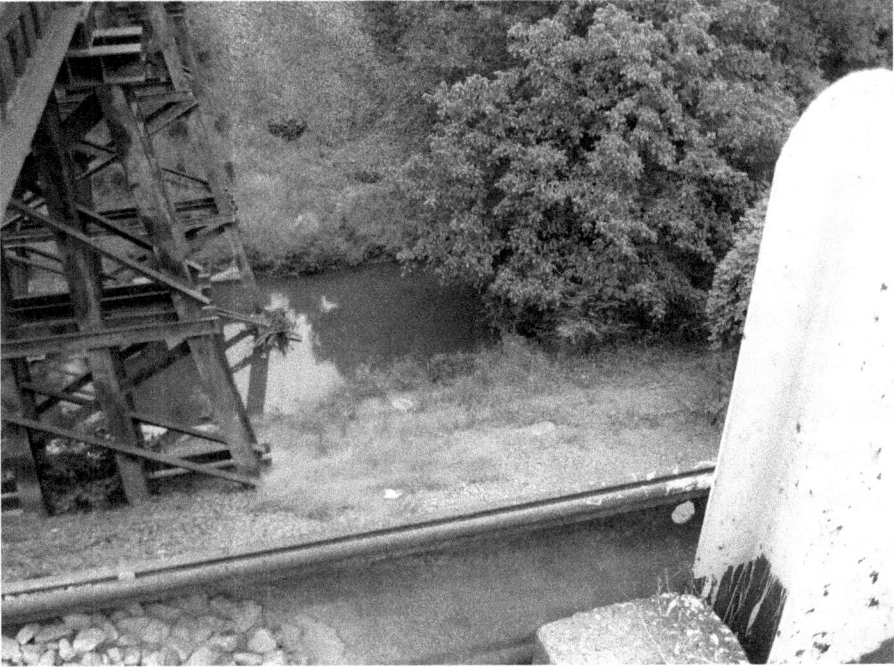

The gentle flow of Camp Creek can be seen under the bridge in September 2008.

he felt strong enough, the night would have been an even bigger tragedy. This man's heroism should never be understated. The operator at the McDonough station received orders to hold everything, for there was danger ahead. Quinlan then rounded up as many people as he could to help rescue survivors at the scene. He focused on finding physicians, and a special train was called to carry them to the crash site. Quinlan worked the entire night. He did not return to the crash site until the next morning.[51]

When the rescue effort began, the cars of the train had already caught fire. In addition to braving the swift-moving and deep waters of Camp Creek, the rescuers had to avoid being consumed by the flames. On top of that, the location of the wreck was not ideal for rescue operations. Camp Creek lies two miles north of McDonough and three miles from the station at Flippen. There were only a few houses near the scene of the wreck, one of which was John McDonald's. His home was quite small, so it could not be used as a morgue or a makeshift treatment center for survivors.[52]

Q.A. DICKSON REACHES THE SCENE

The awful location and obstacles did not stop the rescuers, although it did make their work more difficult. Another hero who sprung into action that night was Mr. Q.A. Dickson. Dickson was asleep in his home when the crash occurred, but he was awakened by someone shouting outside his door. When Dickson sprang from his bed to see what the commotion was about, he found a man in his yard yelling and moving about as if he were deranged. This man was J.J. Quinlan. Quinlan had stopped on his way back to McDonough to rouse sleepers and turn them into rescuers. Quinlan told Dickson that there had been a crash. Dickson claimed that Quinlan jumped up and down as he spoke and fidgeted with his hands. He asked Dickson to get help and go to the creek while he went back to McDonough to flag a train. Dickson said that he hesitated for a few seconds, and Quinlan advanced toward him in a threatening manner so as to impress upon him the importance of moving quickly. Dickson was convinced that something was wrong and agreed to get moving.[53]

When Dickson reached the scene, he was horrified at what he saw. Taking in the situation around him, he quickly spotted people standing on top of the sleeper car near the embankment. He told reporters:

> *I think I was the first man to lay eyes on the terrible scene. I took in the situation at a glance and shouted to the men on top of the sleeper. They screamed to me that they could not get out, and asked if I could get a rope. I at once went and got the only one available, which was my plot line, and as I had used it all the season, was afraid it would not hold. When I again reached the wreck several men were standing on the bank. The rope proved stronger than I thought it was, and one after another we pulled them up. One man weighed about two hundred pounds, but he got up all right.[54]*

Dickson kept working, all the while watching the scene of misery and death unfold around him. The coaches and other cars began to incinerate right before his eyes, and the screams of doomed men pierced the night. Apparently, the scene had a profound effect on Dickson, for he said that "unless a person has experienced what I did, unless he has seen people burning to death and being crushed and beaten about, all the while shrieking and crying for help which might as well been ten miles away, that person cannot appreciate what I am saying." He commented further that he hoped God would take him from this earth before he ever had to witness such a sight again.[55]

Jesse Rohr:
A Baltimore Salesman Speaks of the Wreck

Another firsthand witness to the accident was passenger Jesse L. Rohr of Baltimore, a traveling salesman. He, too, was in the Pullman sleeper. He mentioned that the crash happened as suddenly as was reported by the other survivors. There was no kind of warning whatsoever, and the passengers onboard had no idea that there was any kind of danger ahead until it was too late. According to Rohr, the passengers on the Pullman heard a crash and then felt their car lunge forward and drop. At that time, the forward end of the sleeper car started filling up with water, a fact reiterated by the other survivors, including Miss Merritt, Quinlan and Miss Alden. As water poured into the sleeper car, the lights were extinguished, leaving all onboard in total darkness. The roar of rushing water could be heard, and Rohr deduced that they were in some stream or other body of water. This testimony underscores the complete ignorance of the passengers about what had happened.

Rohr got down on his hands and knees, felt around in the darkness and then began climbing to the upper end of the sleeper. This was, in part, to keep himself from being drowned in the rushing water quickly overtaking the car. Finally reaching the end of the sleeper car, he crawled outside. He said that he noticed the car was hanging by its rear trucks from the stone abutment of the culvert, swaying back and forth like a great pendulum in the current. By this time, Rohr said that the rain was coming down hard and the night was dark. The only light was coming from the part of the train that had started to burn, but even that did not do much to pierce the darkness. What struck Rohr the most was the fact that the darkness was not full of cries for help. He realized that the passengers in the other cars must have been killed instantly. By the time he reached the top of the car and gathered himself, the other cars were engulfed in flames. A reporter asked Mr. Rohr about the washout itself—how wide it was—and he replied that he didn't know. To him, it was as wide as the Mississippi, and the roar of the flames and running creek were enough to unnerve anyone.[56]

Other testimony from that fateful night came from C.P. Hightower, an operator at the depot in McDonough when the crash happened. He was seated at his desk expecting Engine #7 to arrive at Atlanta as planned. In his testimony, he, too, mentioned that the rain was pouring down heavily. All was quiet, and there was no activity on any of his instruments. He alluded to the fact that a strange feeling overtook him about forty minutes after #7 had left McDonough. The silence of the evening was broken when he heard someone running up to the station. He knew at that point that something was wrong. Before he could answer the door, a figure covered with mud from head to toe and showing signs of bleeding appeared at the door. The man was gasping for breath and soaking wet. The man, whom we now know was J.J. Quinlan, yelled, "For God's sake, hold that train! Number 7 is in the creek burning up!" After that, Quinlan collapsed. Hightower, realizing that he had to stop the freight train, ran out to the platform and flagged the train as it was just pulling in. At that point, Hightower worked to secure a car on the incoming freight train to send supplies and rescue workers to the scene of the Camp Creek crash.[57]

Around midnight, a wrecking train was sent to the sight of the crash. However, the burning wreck prevented any real work from happening at the site. The next day, at 6:00 a.m., a special train was dispatched, transporting doctors, ministers, railroad officials and helpers to the scene. But there was not much that could be done, except gather the bodies of the victims still left at the site.[58]

As would be expected, doctors were needed on the scene, and right after J.J. Quinlan reached the depot in McDonough, rescue workers were recruited and a train was dispatched. Doctors were rounded up to be sent to the site, including C.D. McDonald and D.W. Scott. Early arrivals to the scene mentioned that the coaches were already on fire, and the light from

The Heroes

HORROR OF HORRORS!

Wild Plunge of a Passenger Train Into Camp Creek Culvert.

Left: An article that ran in the *Henry County Weekly* on June 29, 1900, about the crash.

Below: A copy of an article in the *Atlanta Constitution* about the crash.

THIRTY-ONE LIVES LOST IN M'DONOUGH DISASTER; GREATEST LIFE LOSS KNOWN IN SOUTHERN WRECK

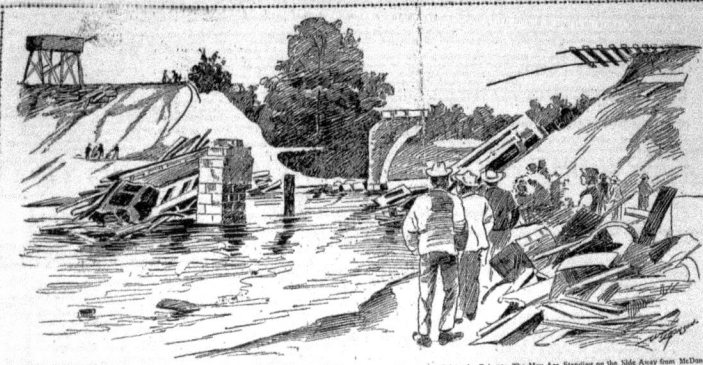

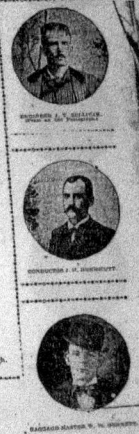

BY DANIEL GAREY.

the flames illuminated the area enough to see the passengers gathered on top of the sleeper car. It was those passengers who were helped by Q.A. Dickson and pulled to safety one by one with his rope. News of the wreck spread very quickly through the area, and throngs of locals began to arrive. They lined the banks of the creek to do what they could.[59]

CHAPTER SIX

VICTIMS AND SURVIVORS

As day broke, the rescuers noticed that the waters of Camp Creek were starting to recede. This made it more possible to start retrieving the bodies of victims. The body of D.Y. Griffith, a railroad supervisor, was found over a mile from the scene, obviously carried downstream by the raging waters of the creek. J.E. Wood, who had been alive when John McDonald reached him, died on the banks of the creek. His body was recovered from there. Oscar Ellis, a bridge laborer from Stockbridge, was also alive when rescuers reached him, but his body was so mangled that he died later of his injuries. Oddly enough, based on testimony given by those who were in the sleeper car, as well as those who found his body, J.T. Sullivan, the engineer, appeared to have made an attempt to save himself by jumping out of the engine. His body was found some distance from the wreck. Rescuers theorized that had he remained in the engine and not tried to jump, he would have suffered an even more gruesome death, for he would have been penned in and burned alive.

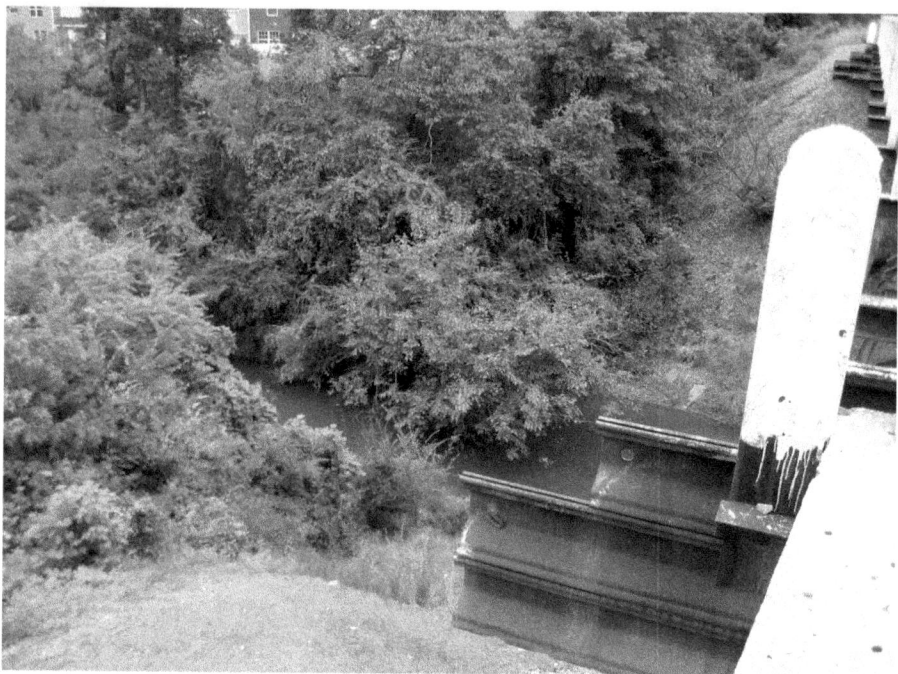

A view of Camp Creek as seen from the bridge where the crash occurred.

The Mystery of the Woman and Her Baby

Stories circulated about a woman who may or may not have been on the train when it crashed. Some said that she was onboard when the train left McDonough, but others mentioned that they thought she had gotten off in Jackson. Those who saw her board the train said that she was carrying a baby. When survivors and rescuers were interviewed after the crash and during the rescue operation, some of them reported seeing a woman floating downstream, screaming for help. It was also reported that a lady's hat and a baby's diaper were found down the creek from the wreck. The diaper had a baby pin in it, indicating that it had washed off the body of a child.[60]

In addition, the *Atlanta Constitution* reported that rescuers saw the body of a baby and its mother on the banks of the creek, but moments later, the two were swept away, never to be seen again. Their bodies were never recovered.[61] Other reports from the same paper, released on the same day, reported that no women were killed on the train.[62] A few days later, the *Macon Telegraph* reported that there was no woman in the day coach with a baby when the train crashed. A Mr. Banks reported that there was a woman and a little boy who departed the train at Jackson and that was the last woman in the day coach. The only other women onboard were Miss Merritt and Miss Alden.[63] But questions still remain: Why did the rescuers report seeing a woman and baby lifeless on the creek bank and then washed downstream? Were they delirious from their work, or is it possible that there was another woman onboard in another car? Perhaps we will never know if this woman was involved in the crash. Several bodies were never recovered, and it might be that she and her baby were two of them.

RECOVERING BODIES

As the morning continued, rescuers worked hard to recover bodies that might have been carried off by the creek. Four bodies were found lying underneath the debris that had collected under the washout. They were burned beyond recognition, but one of them was thought to be Fireman Ed Bird. Among the rescuers who worked all night and into the next day were Q.A. Dickson, who, as mentioned before, helped pull survivors off the top of the sleeper with a rope; Henry County Sheriff Glass; Dr. McDonald; A.F. Bunn; Jack Nolan; A.A. Lemmon; J.B. Newman; S.J. Brown; Reverend F.S. Hudson; and W.H. Barnett. Q.A. Dickson led the search parties since he was so familiar with the layout of the area. The search crews carried picks, shovels and rope to clear away timbers and other items from the wreck.

About a mile down creek from the wreck, wreckage and other debris washed up and were caught in a bend. It all began to pile up in that one place, and a terrible stench arose. At first, rescuers and cleanup crews thought that there might be bodies lodged in the mass, but upon further examination, there were no bodies or body parts. The stench seemed to have been created from all the foliage and vegetation that had accumulated there. It did, however, draw a large crowd of curious onlookers. One rescuer commented that the stench was compounded by the hot, sweltering sun and the presence of green flies swarming everywhere.[64] It is important to keep in mind that these rescuers and search parties were doing their work in the midst of the hot Georgia summer. In addition, the rains had made everything humid. The ground was soggy, and the workers had to tromp across land that had been underwater when Camp Creek swelled to the size of a small river. It would be very difficult to do usual work in these conditions, much less search for bodies in hopes of finding victims.

As the next few days passed, the rain moved out, and the weather was more conducive to working at the wreck site. Thousands of people visited the wreck in those days. As news of the tragedy spread throughout the area, it was something of a sightseeing venture to go to the wreck to view what was left and try to understand what had happened. Letters, telegrams and other communications began to pour into the Southern Railway offices from family members of the victims, as well as well-wishers who wanted to herald the rescue operation and congratulate those who had made every effort to save survivors from the roof of the Pullman car.

There were some macabre happenings associated with the rescue. It was reported that some rescue workers went through the clothing of the deceased to see what they could find.[65] This enraged many people and caused rumor to spread. Not all of the bodies were desecrated in this way. Rumor circulated that when William A. Barclay's body was taken to the undertaker, it had been robbed. It was later discovered that Barclay had left $200 and a watch with a diamond stud in a safe at the Macon depot. He had not been robbed, but had he not stored those valuables in the safe at Macon, he very well could have been.[66]

⸺⣿⣿⣿⣿⣿⸺

BODIES AND FUNERALS

Another macabre event surrounding the rescue and distribution of remains occurred in McDonough itself, specifically at the city cemetery. According to a report in the *Macon Telegraph*:

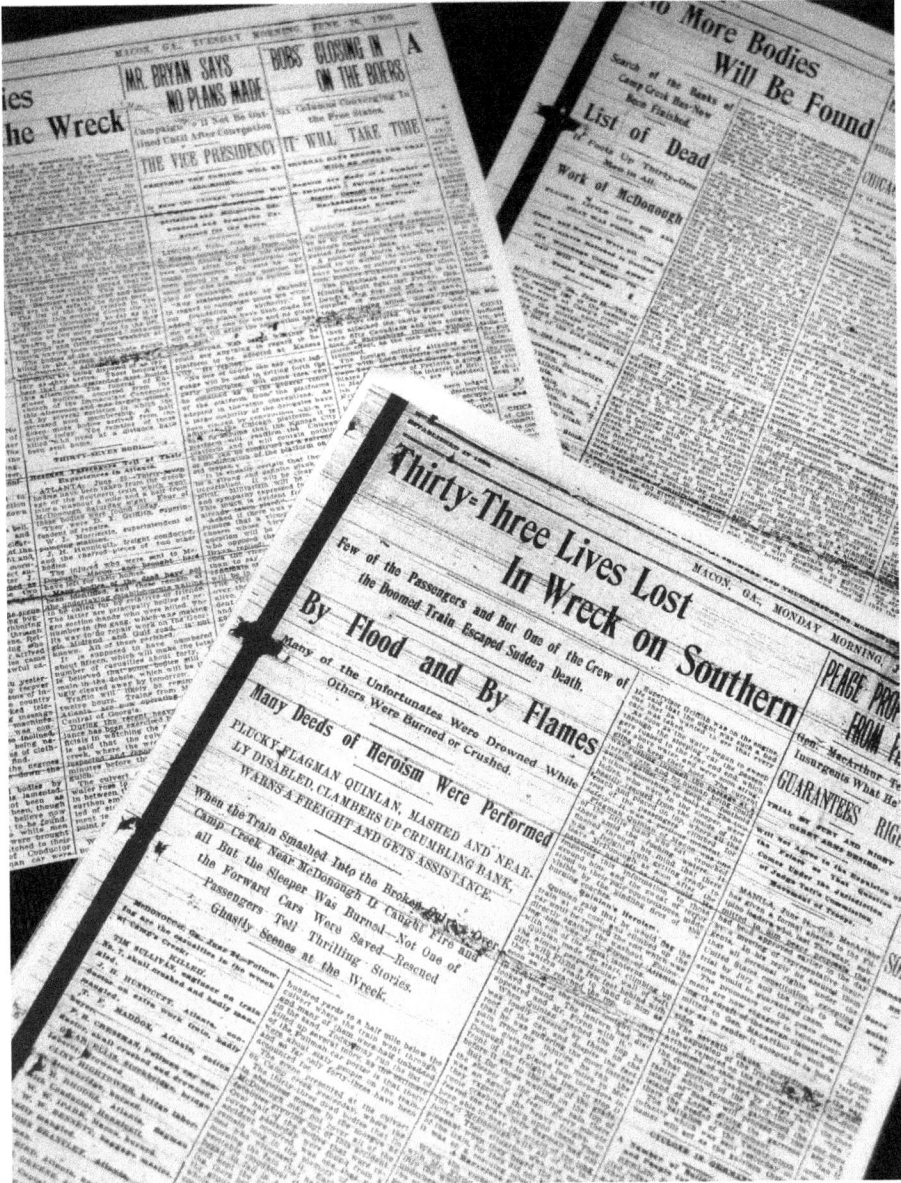

Copies of articles that ran in the *Macon Telegraph* about the crash.

The funeral services over the unrecognizable masses of buried flesh were conducted at the McDonough cemetery today by Rev. F.S. Hudson in the presence of a large crowd. The two shapes supposed to be whites were buried separately. The scene was a particularly impressive one, and women wept for those beings being interred in the unknown graves.[67]

Today, there is a statue of a woman holding a baby in the center of the McDonough Memorial Cemetery. Local rumor circulates that this woman and her child died in the train crash. However, there is no record that they were passengers on the train. Additionally, their dates of death are listed as over a year after the crash occurred. This is an example of how local legends get started and never die. However, since the name on the tombstone was the name of a very prominent family in McDonough, and this stone is located in that family's plot, it would be entirely logical to assume that some report or record of this woman and her child would have circulated. No names have ever been connected to the bodies of the woman and child that some rescuers allegedly saw in Camp Creek, certainly not the names of the woman and child listed on that stone in the cemetery.

Many of the bodies that were recovered from the crash were taken back to McDonough, as that was the closest city with funeral home establishments. However, at the time of the crash, there were only two funeral homes in McDonough. They were B.B. Carmichael & Sons and A.F. Bunn & Company. Both funeral homes were located in downtown McDonough, and both were very prominent businesses in the community. Oddly, these two funeral homes were also furniture companies. The bodies were divided between the homes for preparation. Neither facility could accommodate that many dead, so some of the corpses were placed in coffins and laid out in the square in downtown McDonough to await removal. There has been some debate and discussion about this, with some researchers saying that there was no proof of this. However, in Vessie Thrasher Rainer's *Henry County, Georgia: The Mother of Counties*, Mrs. Rainer quotes a newspaper article in which C.G. Alexander comments that he did not think he would ever forget the sight of all those coffins lined up around the square.[68]

It is not clear how many bodies were brought to the square. It appears that several unidentified bodies were not brought there but were buried on the banks of Camp Creek, not far from the wreck site. According to an article in the *Atlanta Constitution* from July 12, 1900, a man named John Brantley was finally identified by his wife. However, the story of how he

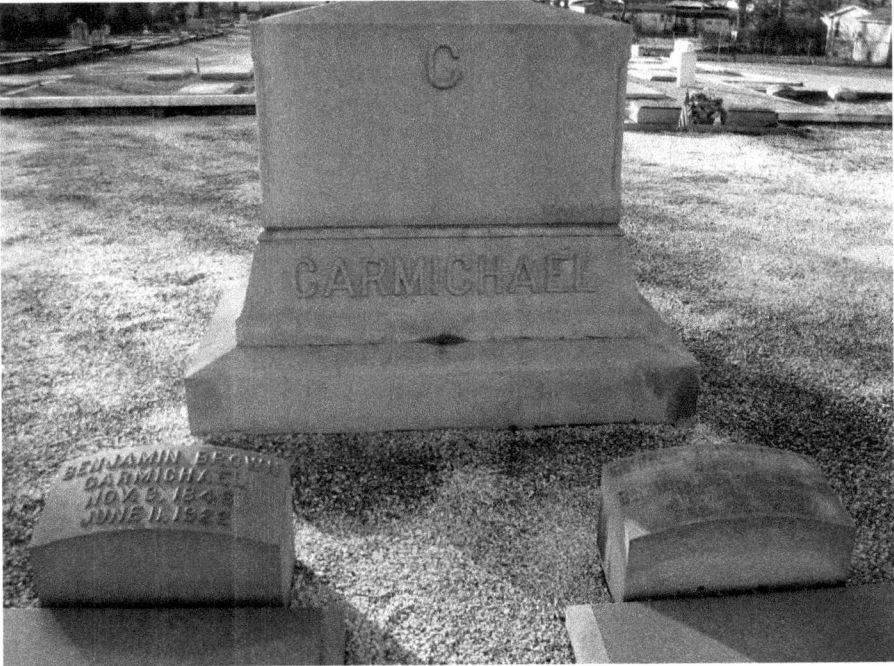

The grave of undertaker B.B. Carmichael, one of the undertakers who prepared bodies of the victims on the night of the crash.

was identified was quite odd and almost reads like a scene from a horror film. The article reports:

> *Nearly three weeks after the frightful wreck on the Southern Railway near McDonough the body of John Brantley was exhumed from one of the graves of the unknown yesterday and was brought to Atlanta last night. A young wife and an anxious family and many other relatives waited to hear tidings of him, and as the days passed by and no news was received from him, the belief that he was among the killed in the wreck gained credence, and yesterday it was decided to exhume the bodies of the unknown. Yesterday morning Undertaker C.H. Swift, accompanied by a brother of the missing man, went to Camp Creek and all four of the graves marked unknown were opened. In one of them a body was found which was identified as that of John Brantley. The head was gone and one arm and a leg were torn off, but a burn on the body and a scar on the remaining hand served to show that the body was that of John Brantley.[69]*

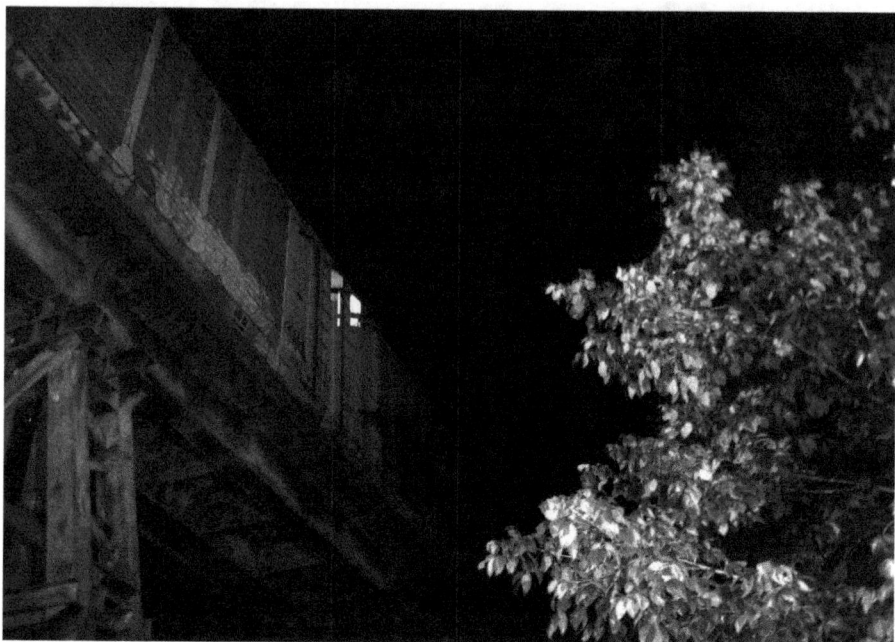

A train passes over Camp Creek on June 23, 2009, the 109th anniversary of the crash. The track is still an active track.

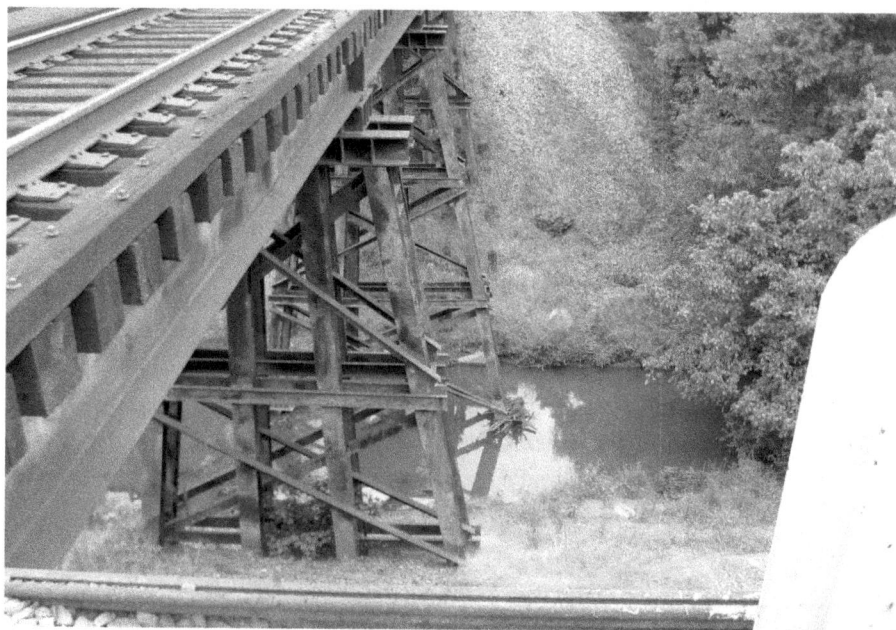

A view of the creek from the current bridge.

There has been no other mention of bodies buried at the site of the wreck on the banks of Camp Creek. However, it would be hard to imagine that the *Atlanta Constitution* would print a story with absolutely no foundation or in which the reporter had no verification whatsoever. Curiosity-seekers, tour guides and historians have visited the site of the crash since it occurred in 1900. Each year, on the anniversary of the wreck, a local tour guide conducts a tour of the area at the hour of the crash. The group waits until a train from the local depot moves overhead. Little do they know that the remains of some of the victims of that wreck may very well be right under their feet.

THE DEAD GO HOME

The crashed train carried quite a few people from Atlanta, especially the crew. By Monday evening, trains that had been dispatched to pick up the remains of the dead from Atlanta began arriving there. On Monday night, June 24, two trains carrying eight dead pulled into the depot. Crowds had already assembled at Peters Street Crossing to see the sight. The train carried the bodies of William A. Barclay, a conductor and the engineer, James T. (J.T.) Sullivan. Two other bodies, those of D.C. Hightower and W.O. Ellis, both of whom were Southern Railway employees, were taken to Stockbridge. It was estimated that over fifteen hundred people turned out to see the spectacle. The second train that arrived at the Peters Street Crossing carried the bodies of W.J. Pate and, perhaps the most devastating loss of the crash, his thirteen-year-old son. Also on that train were the bodies of W.F. Maddox and William Green, a fireman on the train crew, as well as two conductors, H.R. Cressman and J.E. Woods, whom John McDonald had tried to save. Later, a third train arrived in Atlanta carrying the bodies of George W. Flournoy and Conductor J.H. Hunnicutt, both of Atlanta.[70]

A report in the *Atlanta Constitution* described the scene at the Peters Street Crossing on the night of the first train's arrival:

The crowd at Peters Street crossing gathered before 8 o'clock last night. No one seems to have informed the crowd that the bodies would be taken off at that point, but the people came on as by intuitive instinct. Presently the wagons of the funeral directors drove up to the crossing and waited and the curious crowd was convinced. It rained meantime and the torches of the dusky train men as they ran here and there across the wide area of track lit up the place with a fitful and death-like glamour. When a switch engine came by, forced to slow up by the great element of danger, the crowd made a wild dive at it, peering in to see if by any chance it carried dead bodies. Finally the dead came and the people had to be driven back with police club to keep them from interfering with the undertakers and their work. There were in the big crowd the sisters and wives of the men known to have been or thought to be in the terrible wreck; their brothers and their friends mingled here and there in the curious mob that demanded for the time being a sight of death.[71]

Conductor William A. Barclay was taken to Atlanta at first, but soon afterward, his body was taken to Selma, Alabama. According to reports, his funeral was one of the largest ones held in Selma. Businesses in the soon-to-be-famous Alabama town were closed for the services. It appears that his funeral procession passed through the heart of the town, where many local citizens turned out to pay their respects. Condolences and floral arrangements were sent from all over the South.[72] Barclay was thirty-two years old when he was killed in the crash. He was living in Atlanta with his wife and his three-year-old daughter at the time, and he had been with Southern Railway for quite a few years. He was a member of the Macon Division of the Order of Railway Conductors.[73]

James T. Sullivan, the engineer, was buried in Oakland Cemetery. The sexton at the cemetery has no record of the burial, but several obituaries indicate that he is buried there. Sullivan was the husband of Mrs. Lizzie Sullivan, formerly Miss Lizzie Malone. The Malone family, one of the early families of Atlanta, has a large plot at Oakland, and many members of that family are interred there, including Thomas J. Malone, Mrs. Sullivan's father, who came to America from Ireland and eventually settled with his family in Atlanta. He became one of the city's tax assessors.[74] Thomas J. Malone is buried at Oakland Cemetery in Lot 545. According to Oakland records, two members of the Sullivan family are buried with him—T.M. Sullivan, who died in 1917, and Mrs. E. Sullivan, who died in 1928.[75] Many believe that James T. Sullivan is buried in this same plot, although his place of burial and any record of it have not been located. Sullivan's funeral was held at the Church of the Immaculate Conception at 3:30 p.m. on June 25, 1900. The end of his obituary, like all the other articles mentioning his interment, clearly states that his burial was at Oakland Cemetery.[76]

Sadly, Mrs. Sullivan was expecting her husband home that evening and even went so far as to prepare him a special meal at their residence in Atlanta at 698 South Pryor Street. Since the weather was stormy, she knew that her husband would arrive home wet and hungry. She baked fresh bread, which she made sure was done baking right about the time that her husband's train would be arriving in Atlanta. Sullivan should not have been the engineer that evening. He was a replacement for another engineer, James T. Pittman. Pittman's daughter had taken ill, some say with pneumonia, and Sullivan graciously agreed to take his place on the Macon to Atlanta run, a decision that led to his death.

Most everyone felt confident in Sullivan's ability to drive a train, but the conditions that night, and the damage done to the culvert that held up the tracks and bridge over Camp Creek, made Sullivan's skills irrelevant. No engineer could have piloted his train across that bridge safely. Sullivan not only left behind a good wife but he also left behind six children. Mrs. Sullivan was aboard the train that brought her husband's body back to Atlanta at the Peters Street Crossing.[77] Another interesting fact about Mr. Sullivan is that his sister married J.J. Haverty, founder of Haverty's Furniture Company, which still operates in over 120 locations across seventeen states today.[78]

The body of J.E. Wood was also brought to Atlanta on the second train that arrived at Peters Street Crossing. Wood resided on Mills Street in Atlanta at the time of his death. He was forty-nine years old, and like Sullivan, he left behind a wife. She was left to care for three children alone. Wood was not supposed to return to Atlanta until midweek; however, he made the trip early so that he could spend Sunday with his family. Other Atlantans who died on the wreck include W.W. Bennett, W.W. Iparks, J.H. Hunnicutt and William H. Green. Bennett was a baggage master who resided on Woodward Avenue. Sadly, at his death, he left behind not only a widow but also a newborn baby. He was originally from Augusta, which is where his parents resided at the time of his death. He was on the rise at Southern Railway, having just been promoted to the position he held at the time of the crash.[79]

W.W. Iparks was a new resident of Atlanta, having moved there from Richmond, Virginia, just before the crash. He resided on Houston Street with his wife and his four-year-old son. It was reported that neither he nor his wife had any living relatives. His father had died when he was just four years old. He was a prominent businessman, with many contacts throughout the southeastern United States. J.H. Hunnicutt, also a conductor, lived in Atlanta on Luckie Street—quite an ironic name given the way he died. A prominent figure within the railroad industry, he, too, was a member of the Order of Railway Conductors. He was forty years old at the time of his death, and like the others, he left a widow. He had no children, however. He was buried at Oakland Cemetery in a Masonic ceremony. William H. Green was a fireman onboard the ill-fated train. He was a bit younger than the others, who were part of the railroad's crew from Atlanta, only having reached the age of twenty-three by the time of the crash. He was returning to Atlanta to spend Sunday with his mother. Having recently moved to Atlanta from Columbus, Georgia, Green lived on Whitehall Street. He was survived by two brothers, five sisters and his mother. His body was returned to Columbus for burial.[80]

As the train originated in Macon, naturally there were a number of people onboard who lived there and whose bodies were taken back to that city. Several of these were railroad employees, as was the case in Atlanta. The remains of J.H. Rhodes were brought to Macon to await transportation to a small community called Alcorn, near the Washington County town of Tennille. His body had already been prepared for burial in McDonough, and his brother and sister came to Macon to retrieve it. Stricken with grief, both siblings asked for the coffin to be opened so that they could see their departed loved one's face one more time; however, those who brought the body back to Macon labored hard to dissuade the two from doing so because they knew how horrifying it would be to see the badly mutilated remains of their brother. The two agreed, and they asked the undertaker to seal the coffin for good before they proceeded to Alcorn.[81]

The remains of W.L. Morrisette were also brought back to Macon. Morrisette was from Pocahontas, Virginia, but worked for the Southern Railway as a pump agent. He was very active in the Masonic Lodge in Macon, and due to the fact that his family was mainly in Virginia, his lodge brothers took care of his remains under instruction from his sister. The remains were taken to Keating's funeral establishment, where they were kept until they could be transported by train to Midlothian, a suburb of Richmond. The night before they were sent out, hundreds of friends and fellow Masons came to the undertaker's to view them. Although the head and face were crushed badly, the morticians in McDonough had repaired them enough so that Morrisette could be identified. Other remains that were brought to

Macon included those of Clay Franks, a railroad employee; Flagman W.H. Green, who had already been taken to Atlanta but was sent back through Macon on his way to Columbus for burial; and W.J. Pate and his thirteen-year-old son, Jesse, who were being sent to Griffin for burial.[82]

Also in Macon, rumors circulated that Deputy Marshall George F. White might have been on the train when it crashed. However, Mr. White soon appeared on the scene to dispel that rumor. He recounted that he and Cliff Vigal were on the train, but they disembarked at Jackson, where they were to make a raid. He gave no further details about the raid, but he did recount a very interesting story about J.C. Flynn, a passenger on the train who survived. It appears that as the two, White and Vigal, boarded the train, they sat with Flynn in the smoking car, where they laughed and talked about different things. At some point on the ride from Macon to Jackson, Flynn started talking about the fact that he had about $2,000 with him on the trip. Almost prophetically, Flynn commented that it was a bad night for traveling and that even if it cost him a fourth of what he had on him in cash, he thought he would go back to the sleeper car, where he would be safer. Marshall White went on to say:

> *When I heard of the wreck at 5 o'clock Sunday morning, I went up to McDonough and saw Jack. He said this was the fourth wreck he had been in within a year, and if he lived to get to Atlanta this time, he thought he would stay there and quit traveling as luck seemed to be against him. I thought luck was with him, for when he fell off that sleeper with the lantern in his hand he went entirely under the sleeper and the torrent washed him out. He was carried fully a mile down the stream. Any other man would have been drowned I believe. He did not think of his $2000.00 until Sunday at dinner, when he felt for it and found it all right. He escaped just as miraculously in the Nancy Hanks wreck up here near Summerfield a few years ago, and his life was spared in the Michigan wreck, so it looks as though he can pull through all right wherever you put him.[83]*

It appears that J.C. Flynn was quite lucky. His story, more so than that of any other survivor of the wreck, was impressive. As the old saying goes, "It is the stuff of legends." J.C. Flynn was the last survivor of the Camp Creek crash to pass away. He never forgot the tragic evening he spent in McDonough in 1900. Eventually, he moved to Mt. Vernon, New York, and on December 11, 1958, he made his last visit to the city.[84] Deputy Marshall White was right on the mark with his assessment that Flynn was quite lucky.

He not only survived two train wrecks before the one at Camp Creek, but he also survived everyone associated with the Camp Creek wreck.

Another twist to the Camp Creek wreck was reported by noted Henry County historian Vessie Thrasher Rainer in *Henry County, Georgia: The Mother of Counties* (1971). In her book, Mrs. Rainer writes:

> *In the progress of the work at the Camp Creek trestle, two feet were found imbedded under it last week, and upon investigation were identified as those of Clinton Hightower by means of the shoes he wore. They were taken to Stockbridge by his parents and interred with the body.*[85]

This story is oftentimes recounted on the tours given by Dan Brooks and Caprice Walker in McDonough. One tour participant, upon hearing this, leaned over to ask another participant if he thought it was true. Responding to this, an older lady leaned over and replied to the two, "Yes, it actually is. I have read that before in an old Henry County newspaper. Besides, that kind of thing is just too good to make up." She was right. The story was printed in the August 31, 1900 edition of the *Henry County Weekly*. It must also be noted that the elderly tour participant was on to something in her assessment that the story of Hightower's feet was just too good to make up. In fact, many people, upon hearing some of the stories researchers like myself have found, comment that these kinds of tales are great examples of instances where fact is just stranger than fiction.

SURVIVORS AND THE "MAYBE" DEAD

For a short time after the wreck, there was a great deal of debate about a few people who might have been on the train when it wrecked, much like the speculation about Deputy Marshall White. The strangest of these stories concerns two men, one named Jensen and the other named Caprelian. It appears in several articles about the wreck, including a few secondary pieces written as of late, that there was a W.H. Jenson onboard the doomed train when it wrecked at Camp Creek. Early reports included his name, and there was even an attempt to contact his relatives to identify the remains and retrieve them. The problem was that he was alive, and the remains that needed retrieving were not his. In fact, the remains were of a man named Caprelian (last name), and he was a traveler from New York. It was not stated if he was a traveling salesman, and it is entirely possible that he could have been on vacation or just a world traveler seeing different parts of the country.

In an interesting turn of events, when the body was thought to be that of W.H. Jenson, a Mormon elder from Sugar, Utah, it was Mr. Jensen himself who corrected that mistake. After the correction was made concerning Mr. Jenson, a proper identification did not quickly come. In fact, one Elder Sorrensen of the Mormon Church incorrectly identified the body as that of a man named Bennisen. However, another leader in the Mormon Church from Chattanooga verified that there was no one in the Mormon Church in Georgia by that name. That leader, a man identified as President Rich, came to Georgia personally to identify the body but failed. After additional research, the body was correctly identified as that of Mr. Caprelian, but no further information about his identity or what he was doing traveling through Georgia was produced.[86]

In addition to the misidentification of Mr. Caprelian's body, W.W. Zapp was thought to be onboard the train. The article in the *Atlanta Constitution* that carried the story reported that "he declines positively to be dead." While this was an interesting way of declaring Mr. Zapp's condition, the important thing was that this eliminated his name from the list of victims.[87] Others who were thought to be on the ill-fated train were J.T. Buchanan of Atlanta, who was reportedly missing. He eventually received word that he was associated with the list of victims of the train and eagerly made his presence, and the fact that he was very much alive, known to his brother-in-law, J.F. White. He was doing quite well and working in Southwest Georgia. He further reported that he was supposed to be on the train but had decided at the last minute to stay in Southwest Georgia and finish his work before returning home to Atlanta, perhaps a decision that saved his life. In addition, an A.W. McClellan, who was also in the Southwest Georgia area when the crash happened, was thought by his family to have been a passenger on the train when it crashed. However, shortly afterward, he was located in Florida. He telegraphed his family to relay that he was safe in Florida as soon as he heard that there was speculation that he was one of the victims.[88]

J.J. Quinlan, whose real name was Johnnie, was perhaps the best known of all the survivors and the one who is credited with great acts of heroism. After his efforts to stop the freight train from barreling down the tracks and crashing on top of the already burning mass, as well as his efforts to save the survivors from peril, he was examined for injuries. His neck was badly swollen and his back was quite sore.[89]

On the lighter side of such a dark episode, a story was told in Macon of a young man who was quite well-known in his community. He purchased a ticket on the doomed train for a trip to Atlanta. However, and luckily, the young man's friends asked him to wait in Macon and delay his trip to the capital city. He refused their pleas. Not to be discouraged, his friends promised that they would treat him to a barbecue and a night of cards if he stayed. He agreed and remained in Macon. It turns out that he won eleven dollars in the card game. He commented that he was "satisfied that there is nothing immoral in cards because this game certainly saved his life."[90] It would probably be difficult to find anyone who would disagree with that sentiment.

CHAPTER SEVEN

THE AFTERMATH

After the wreck, various reports began to surface alluding to the sordid history of Old Engine #7. According to these reports, the engine had had more than its fair share of catastrophes. In fact, the engine had already spent some time in the bed of another creek.

The engine was put into service in 1888 by the Southern Railway Company. That year, the train claimed its first victims between the towns of Knoxville and Lenoir, Tennessee. It plowed into a farm wagon on the tracks and killed three people. Ten years later, in 1897, the same engine took another nine lives when it hit a covered wagon carrying members of a local family named Woodward near the city of Avondale, right outside of Chattanooga, Tennessee. It was after this episode that the railroad company decided that it might be best to rename the engine, for fear that it might be cursed or, at minimum, to help allay apprehensions about the history of the machine.

At that point, the number on the engine was 846 (in some articles, 836). The engine was renumbered 851. Apparently, the new number did nothing to stop the death spree, for in 1898, the locomotive made its first dive into a river. According to reports in the *Atlanta Constitution* in July 1900, the rechristened locomotive crashed into a chasm of over sixty feet and landed in the Etowah River. The freight cars attached to the engine caught fire and were destroyed, along with a great deal of freight. Like at Camp Creek on June 23, 1900, rains had swollen the Etowah River and caused damage to the bridge. After that crash, #851 lay buried in the mud of the Etowah for several weeks. According to a report of the incident:

*It was finally raised by the aid of a monster-derrick and a ten wheel
locomotive...It was rebuilt, and sent again on its career of killing, behaving
well until it culminated in the Camp Creek affair. The original number
846 had been restored after raising it from the Etowah.*[91]

The first engineer who drove the 846, John Ramsey, met an untimely
demise when he was scalded to death in an accident stemming from his
work on the engine. As if that were not enough, the second engineer, Abe
Laird, died of typhoid fever during the summer of 1899, just one year
prior to the accident at Camp Creek and one year after the wreck at the
Etowah River. In addition, J.T. Sullivan was the replacement engineer for
James T. Pittman on the night of the crash. From the history of this engine,
one might infer that bad luck followed Old #7 up the track from Macon to
McDonough that night. There are more than just a couple quirks of fate
in the history of this train.[92]

As might be expected, public discussion soon turned to the cause of the
wreck. Soon after the crash, railroad officials publicly acknowledged that
they were investigating the causes of the wreck and what could be done
to prevent further tragedy. At first, the consensus was that there was very
little, if anything, that the railroad company could have done to prevent the
accident. Railroad workers, including John A. McDonald, a man who was
one of the first rescuers on the scene the night of the crash, discussed what
they had seen prior to the crash.

According to McDonald, who at that time was in charge of the pumping
station at Camp Creek, he was working that evening and left just thirty
minutes prior to the crash. He reported that he never saw or heard anything
that would have led him to feel that the approaching trains were in danger.
In addition, the section foreman for the line, a Mr. Croxdale, reported that
there was not one thing that led him to think there might be a catastrophe
that evening. Croxdale, like McDonald, had been in the vicinity of Camp
Creek that day. According to Croxdale, the culvert was constructed in such a
way that no engineer would have thought it possible for water—any amount
of water—to compromise the bridge and endanger the track.[93] Apparently,
the danger was hidden but very present.

Soon, the officials at the Southern Railway Company became more guarded
in their statements about the wreck. When questioned, Superintendent
Vaughn, of the Atlanta division, reported that he had no knowledge of
the details of the crash. Macon superintendent A. Gordon Jones was more
helpful, but he prefaced his comments with high praise for Southern Railway

employee Johnnie (J.J.) Quinlan. He further commented that the accident had most certainly resulted from the torrential rainfall that had plagued the area in the weeks before the crash. In his estimation, the water rushed with such force and pressure against the brick culverts that it compromised them, washing part of them away. This was unknown to those who were in charge of that part of the Macon to Atlanta line; therefore, there was no way to let Hightower at the McDonough depot know that approaching trains should be flagged and held at the station.[94]

Upon examination, it was found that the construction of the culvert was beyond defect. The culvert measured about forty feet wide, and on top of it rested an embankment of dirt about fifty feet high. As the waters pushed away the brick culvert, they began to wash away the dirt embankment. When the engine came upon the track at that point, the supports gave way and sent the train and all of its cars plunging into the waters below. Superintendent Jones suggested that, since the track where the crash occurred was straight, Sullivan more than likely saw the track ahead but failed to see any danger, as the track had probably not sagged or given way by the time the train arrived. It was also reported that a passenger train had passed over the bridge about 6:00 p.m. that evening from Macon and that nothing out of the ordinary was reported when this occurred.[95]

Later that summer, insurance claims started to be made against the companies that had insured the lives of the men onboard the train. The company that paid out a great deal of insurance claims was the Standard Accident Insurance Company. A report in the *Atlanta Constitution* listed the claims for several of the deceased. It lists D.Y. Griffith, the supervisor, as having a claim of $3,000 paid to his family. The families of J.H. Rhodes, W.W. Bennett and Ed Byrd each received claims of $1,000. A sum of $2,000 was paid to the families of J.E. Wood and J.H. Hunnicutt.[96]

Most tragedies of this nature bring about legal disputes, and this wreck was no exception. The first lawsuits were filed in Henry County Superior Court; however, they were eventually moved to the United States Circuit Court in Atlanta/Fulton County. By February 7, 1901, no fewer than twenty cases had been filed against the Southern Railway Company.[97] One of the lawyers who represented many of the plaintiffs in these suits was Hoke Smith, who became governor of Georgia in 1907 and served until 1909. He was reelected in 1911. In addition to serving as governor of the state, he was appointed secretary of the interior under President Grover Cleveland. He also served a stint in the United States Senate, representing Georgia. He is buried at Oakland Cemetery, not far from some of the victims of the wreck. Smith had made a name for himself as an injury attorney representing works and passengers against major railroad companies.[98]

It seems that crashes like the one at Camp Creek were just the kind of cases he was accustomed to taking. Some of the cases he took turned out to be winners. Many of the lawsuits contended that the Southern Railway Company had been negligent of its duty and failed to keep the roadbed in a proper state. In response to these claims, Charles Battle, an attorney hired by the Southern Railway Company, argued that the culvert and the embankments were designed correctly and were in safe, secure, working order right up to the date of the crash. Nevertheless, the rains that hit the area in the weeks before the incident were nothing more than an act of God, and it would be impossible to hold the Southern Railway Company accountable for such acts. Subsequently, Battle asked that the courts dismiss the cases.[99] They did not. In fact, many of these cases went to trial, and more than a few juries found Southern Railway to be negligent. Monetary awards, which totaled near $27,000, or about $900 per person, were eventually awarded.[100]

One of the earliest suits to be filed was that of Mrs. Mollie D. Florida, widow of J.R. Florida of Nashville, Tennessee. Mrs. Florida brought her suit against the Southern Railway in the amount of $100,000. This was the first damage suit of its kind filed in Georgia for such a large sum. Mrs. Florida filed for such a large amount because her husband had only reached the age of thirty-nine at the time of his death. At that point, he was earning an estimated $6,000 per year as the owner of a successful publishing business. He was also said to be a very prominent businessman and was quite well known across the South for his publishing work. He had just completed a business tour of the South when he took the doomed train to return home. Mrs. Florida argued that the wreck caused by the defective culvert at Camp Creek robbed her husband of his life and future earning potential for his family. She argued that there was a crack that ran east to west in the culvert underneath the tracks. This breach, she felt, was what caused the culvert to be unable to withstand the pressure hurled against it by the waters of the creek. The suit also mentioned that part of the culvert was washed out before the train passed over and that the railroad was negligent in not keeping someone there to watch the trestle and culvert during the heavy rains.[101] Engineers from the Southern Railway Company testified in the company's defense and stated that the culvert was not defective but that it collapsed as a result of the unusual amount of water in the creek from the rains. The company, they said, should not be held liable for such a catastrophe.[102]

Another suit worth mentioning was the case of Bob Spencer. On March 28, 1901, a suit was filed in the United States Court by Annie Spencer against the railroad company in the amount of $5,000. Mrs. Spencer claimed to be the widow of Robert Spencer, a victim of the wreck and an employee of the Southern Railway Company. Annie Spencer stated that she had married Robert when he was just eighteen years old. Interestingly, Mrs. Annie Spencer was not the only Mrs. Spencer to file a claim against the railroad company as the widow of Robert Spencer. It was noted in a report from the *Atlanta Constitution* that there were three other women claiming to be the widow of Robert Spencer and asking for compensation for his untimely death. The article reports:

> *Thus there are four women who claim to be the widow of Spencer. There may be others to be heard from later. Annie Spencer, who sues in court in Macon, is said to have married Spencer when he was only eighteen years old and she has one child by him. A representative of an Atlanta attorney who has the suit of one of the alleged widows in the Atlanta court was in Macon today to examine papers in the suit filed here. It is a coincidence that all the lawyers in the four suits are named Smith.*[103]

No first names are given for the attorneys whose last names were Smith; however, it would be no great leap in logic to think that at least one of those lawyers was Hoke Smith himself.

Sadly, one of the biggest mysteries of the Camp Creek train crash involves a complete list of people who died as a result of the crash. Newspaper reporters at the time pulled as many records as possible from the Southern Railway Company's list of ticketholders and crew who were supposed to be onboard the train, but those records are inconclusive. Reporters worked on gathering lists and finding out names belonging to recovered bodies. A list of survivors was much easier to compile. Newspapers such as the *Atlanta Constitution*, the *Henry County Weekly* and the *Macon Telegraph* all printed names of survivors and victims. But as has been illustrated, some of the bodies were misidentified, as was the case of Mr. Caprelian, who was misidentified as a Mormon elder named W.H. Jensen of Sugar, Utah. The appendix presents a list of those individuals who were survivors or victims of the wreck, as best as can be assembled from sources available at the time.

EPILOGUE

Standing in the square in downtown McDonough at nightfall, the sound of the oncoming train cannot be mistaken. The whistle blows loudly, warning anyone who might be on the track that it is time to move, for the train is coming and danger may be ahead for those not responsive to the whistle. It is important that trains have whistles to warn bystanders that the track is still active and a train is headed in their direction. Train tracks are places where children sometimes play. Hunters sometimes walk the tracks to get deep into the woods in search of game. Those whistles are a good thing.

Sadly, there was no whistle to warn James T. Sullivan and the rest of the crew of Engine #7 that danger was ahead. There was no way to tell the many passengers onboard the train that they were riding to their deaths. Conductor Cressman sat reading his book in the forward end of the Pullman sleeper and never knew that he was at death's front door. Mamie Merritt and Clara Alden sat across from each other chatting, Merritt with needlework on her lap. They heard no whistle of warning. T.C. Carter, the porter whose hip was dislocated by the crash, never had a warning that he was about to be thrust into a life-threatening situation. Johnnie (J.J.) Quinlan heard no warning whistle that told him of the tragedy about to befall him that would also make him a hero.

Ed Bird, onboard the engine, going steadily about his job, received no advance warning that he was about to be burned alive in the very train that earned him his living. Conductor William A. Barclay never heard a whistle. He left his valuables in a safe back at the Macon depot but it was he who needed safe-keeping. Then there was Mr. Rohr, the traveling salesman from Baltimore, passing through Georgia on the Southern Railway line to help make his living, earning money to participate in civic life as a good citizen. There was nothing to warn him that the train he was on would almost take his life.

There was also no warning for the train's engineer, James T. Sullivan. Although he tried to stop the train when he finally noticed that something was wrong at the bridge, his vision—the only thing he could rely on for advanced warning—was not enough on that night. The rain was pouring down in blinding fashion. The night was dark, and the only light was the oil lantern that burned at the front of the engine. The whistle he blew while barreling down the track did nothing for him. The regular engineer, James T. Pittman, must have felt a sense of remorse that his replacement that night also replaced him in death.

It is unfair that readers, over a century later, have more details and know more about the wreck than did the survivors who were onboard the train.

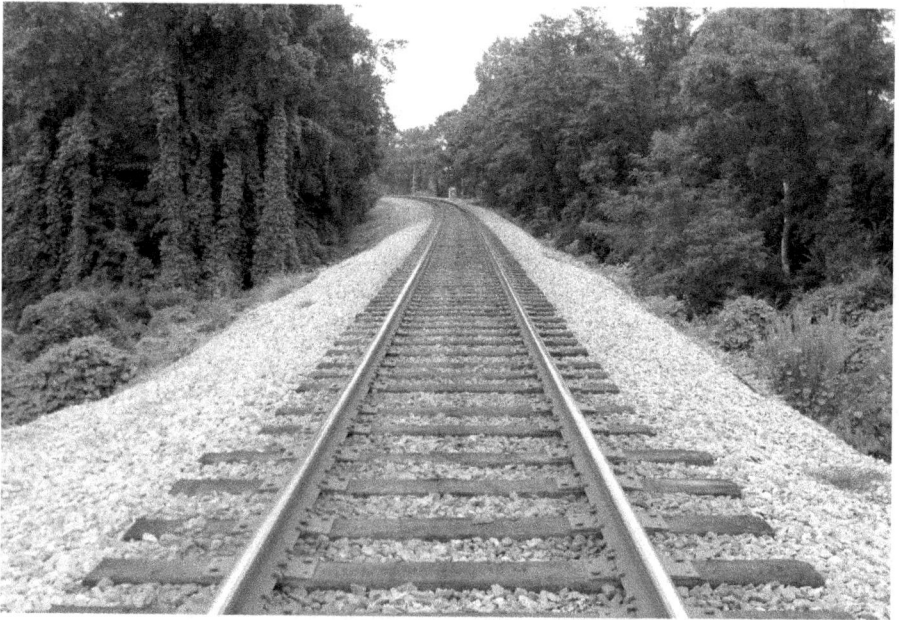

The track that runs north of the crash site today. The train would have taken this route into Atlanta had it not plunged into Camp Creek just a few feet before this run of track.

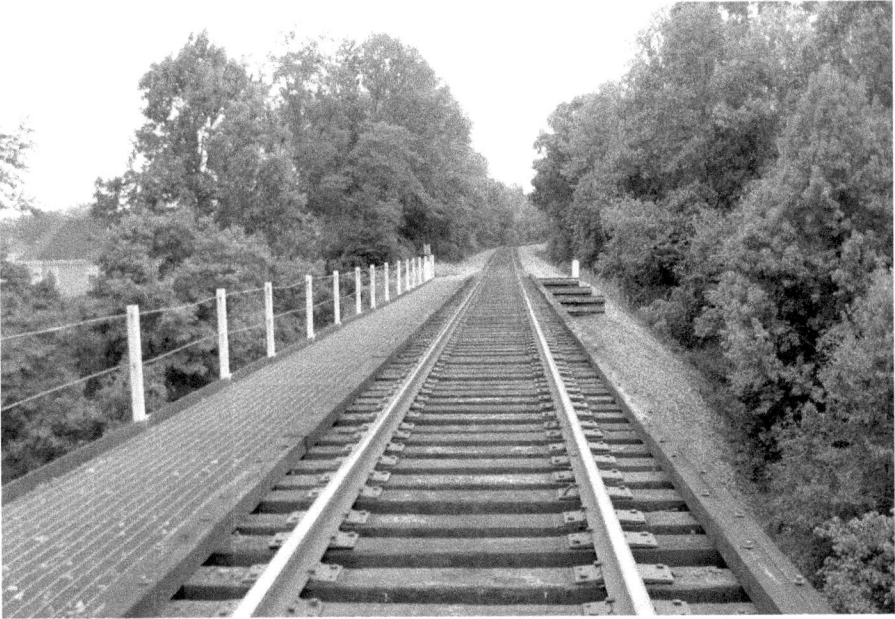

The ill-fated train never crossed the creek on this bridge.

While visitors to the crash site can walk the track today, Old #7 and the cars it pulled never reached that part of the track.

There are many words that can be used to describe the night of June 23, 1900. The crash at Camp Creek was said to be the worst train wreck in the history of Georgia. Of the forty-eight passengers onboard, fewer than a dozen survived. The wreck claimed the lives of almost forty people. They were not all Georgians, either. They came from as far away as Virginia, Utah and Massachusetts. They included men and women, black and white, young and old. Even with limited means of communication, news of the wreck spread like wildfire, and thousands of people came to the small town of McDonough to help with cleanup and search and rescue efforts. The roads and streets of McDonough were as swelled with onlookers and helpers as the Camp Creek was with water on the day of the wreck.

As the days and months passed, so too did the focus on the area and what had happened there. In just a short time, the track was repaired over Camp Creek and rail service resumed, as this was an important thoroughfare for Macon to Atlanta traffic and vice versa. Soon, many of those who were alive in McDonough at the time of the wreck passed away, and automobiles began to replace horses and buggies on the streets of the city. Things changed, as they always do. With the passage of years, the survivors faded one by one. Eventually, Atlanta grew southward, and McDonough, as well as all of Henry County, became part of the thriving South Metro Atlanta area. Interstate 75 was built through the heart of the county, and the growth it brought helped herald many changes to the area. Storefronts sprang up on the roads and highways running through the area, and restaurant and retail store chains dot the landscape where old family businesses once reigned. B.B. Carmichael and Sons is gone; so, too, is A.F. Bunn and Company. The McDonough depot where J.J. Quinlan staggered in, wet, muddy and exhausted, is now the home of a lumber company, and although it still slightly resembles a train depot, most people do not realize its importance in the city's history.

Over time, some in McDonough looked back on the crash as a major happening in the area. Today, there are those who still visit the site of the crash, especially on the anniversary of the wreck. Recently, tour guides Dan Brooks and Caprice Walker started leading tours of the area on June 23 of each year. Fortunately, I was able to attend one of those tours. The night was quiet and unusually cool for June. A crowd of about fifty people assembled at the entrance to the lane that leads to the bank of the creek. Cars were parked all along the road. The tour group made its way down to the creek bank, where Dan discussed the events of that night. Interested onlookers took pictures, climbed the embankments and sat along the banks of the creek, and some brave souls, although chastised by Dan for doing so, managed to climb onto the tracks on the bridge. Visitors explored the creek banks and looked at the brick structures that still remain.

As the night turned dark and the hour of the crash approached, the area fell silent. All that could be heard was the chirping of crickets and the sounds of cars passing by on the roads beside the tracks. The flashes of cameras filled the darkness near the creek. For a few moments, all that the group did was listen, look and wait for the anticipated train to come over the bridge. The train finally arrived, and the noise as it passed overhead was almost unbearable. Nevertheless, the crowd that had assembled felt in some way connected to what happened over one hundred years ago. We had come to the scene, the final destination for almost forty passengers and crew, to explore that connection. We came to memorialize those who died and to honor the heroism of those who worked tirelessly to save the perishing and retrieve the perished.

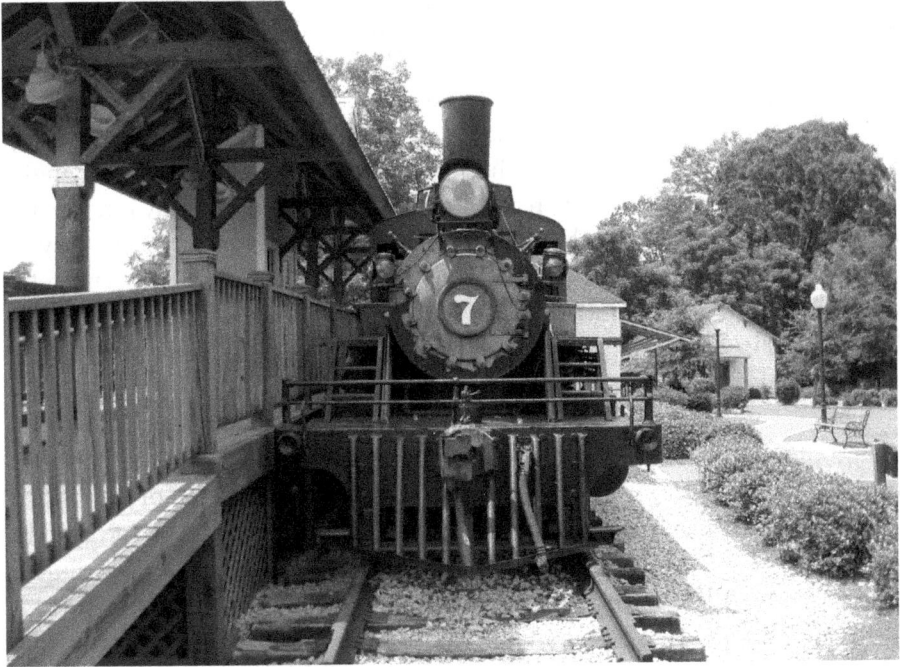

A front view of the replica of Old Engine #7 in Heritage Park in McDonough.

The scene of the wreck is quite different today. While the track is still active and Camp Creek still runs underneath, the waters are certainly not the raging river they were on that night. As a matter of fact, one would need to stand on the creek banks, almost in the water, to hear the trickle of the stream. If you follow the creek upstream just a few hundred feet, it runs across a small road area that trucks and other vehicles apparently cross to access the interior of the forested area where a utility company has equipment. The creek is nothing more than a small stream that could not be responsible for the drowning death of a small wild animal, much less the collapse of an entire bridge and the crash of an engine and its passenger cars. Looking south from the crash site, the rooftops of houses can be seen. There are several new subdivisions that have been built in recent years nearby, one almost on the banks of Camp Creek. The footpaths most certainly made by local children can be seen off to the southeast, leading back to one of the subdivisions. All of this represents the growth and change brought to this area by the more than one hundred years following the doomed passenger train's plunge into the creek. The county-maintained road that leads to the track is also alive and noisy with cars passing by, and farther to the east, Highway 42 connects downtown McDonough with the town of Stockbridge.

Yes, the area has changed a lot since the night of June 23, 1900. The town and county have grown. Those who were alive in McDonough on the night of the crash are now gone. Even the Southern Railway Company is no more, for it was absorbed by the Norfolk Southern Corporation in 1982 and was renamed the Norfolk Southern Railway by 1990. Norfolk Southern is still very active in the area, and its trains continue to run over the Camp Creek bridge, albeit with steel supports instead of the brick culvert that washed away on that stormy June night in 1900.

This is the site of what some have called Georgia's *Titanic*, the place where almost four dozen lives were lost and where widows and orphans were instantly made. It has faded into the bustling landscape of a modern suburb of Atlanta. The night of June 23, 1900, does not stand out to many of the new residents of the area. Although there has been a replica of Old Engine #7 placed on display outside the city at Heritage Park, it serves mostly as a background for curious and climbing children. The most common comments about the history of McDonough among the residents are about how the city and county have grown in the last twenty years to what they are today. People reminisce about how the traffic used to be minimal and the activity that is seen in the shopping malls and retail plazas used to be focused on the square and the downtown area. Although the tracks are still active, the main avenue for traffic through the area is the interstate that connects it to the booming cosmopolitan city of Atlanta. But not far from the interstate runs the track on which Sullivan's engine, blinded by the storm, was headed for breakfast—"in Atlanta or in Hell."

LIST OF SURVIVORS AND VICTIMS

SURVIVORS

Miss Clara Alden, passenger and friend and student of Miss Merritt/
  Boston
T.C. Carter, train porter
Jack C. (J.C.) Flynn, passenger/Flovilla
E.T. Mack, passenger/Chattanooga
Miss Mamie Merritt, passenger and schoolteacher/Boston
Walter Pope, passenger/Atlanta
Johnnie (J.J.) Quinlan, flagman/Macon
Jesse Rohr, passenger/Baltimore
E.S. Schriever, passenger/Chattanooga

(Some papers also mention Handy Tomlinson, but no other information is given about him.)

VICTIMS

W.A. Barclay, conductor/Atlanta
W.W. Bennett, baggage master/Atlanta

Harkness Brady, railroad employee/no city listed
John Brantley, fireman/Atlanta
Ed Byrd, fireman/Tennille
Mr. Caprelian, passenger/New York
H.R. Cressman, conductor/Asheville
John Early, railroad employee/no city listed
W.O. Ellis, bridge laborer/Stockbridge
J.L. Florida, passenger/Nashville, Tennessee
George Flournoy, passenger/Atlanta
Clay Frank, railroad employee/no city listed
W.H. Green, fireman/Atlanta
D.Y. Griffith, division supervisor/Flovilla
Clinton Hightower, passenger/Stockbridge
J.H. Hunnicutt, conductor/Atlanta
W.W. Ipark, passenger/Atlanta
Bob Jester, railroad employee/no city listed
W.R. Lawrence, section foreman/Stockbridge
W.F. Maddox, passenger/Atlanta
W.L. Morrisette, pump repairer/Pocahontas
Jesse Pate, passenger and thirteen-year-old son of W.J. Pate/Atlanta
W.J. Pate, passenger/Atlanta
J.H. Rhodes, flagman/no city listed
Bob Smith, railroad employee/no city listed
Robert Spencer, porter/no city listed
J.T. Sullivan, engineer/Atlanta
J.E. Woods, conductor/Atlanta

(In addition, between ten and eleven unidentified African Americans and whites.)

NOTES

CHAPTER ONE

1. Rainer, *Henry County, Georgia*, 13–14.
2. Sullivan and Georgia Historical Society, *Georgia*, 48.
3. Ibid., 49; and Cook, *Governors of Georgia*, 95.
4. Morris, *True Southerners*, 9.
5. Coulter, *Georgia*, 226.
6. Rainer, *Henry County, Georgia*, 3–4.
7. Ibid., 18.
8. Morris, *True Southerners*, 9.
9. Ibid., 30.
10. Bowen and Turner, *Georgia Confederate Soldiers*, 169–73.
11. Wells, *Moments in McDonough*, 45–48.
12. Bailey, *Chessboard of War*, 48–68.
13. Trudeau, *Southern Storm*, 100–01.
14. Rainer, *Henry County, Georgia*, 283.
15. Speer, *History of Henry County*, 11.

CHAPTER TWO

16 . "Macon & Brunswick Railroad."
17. "East Tennessee, Virginia & Georgia Railroad."

18. Ibid.
19. "Samuel Spencer."
20. "Southern Railway History."
21. *New York Times*, "Samuel Spencer Killed."
22. Rainer, *Henry County, Georgia*, 137.

Chapter Three

23. Sealey, "Camp Creek Wreck."
24. *Atlanta Constitution*, "Inevitable Act of God," 5.
25. Ibid.
26. *Atlanta Constitution*, "Bad Washout," 7.
27. Sealey, "Camp Creek Wreck."
28. *Henry County Weekly*, "Horror of Horrors."
29. Ibid.
30. Brooks and Walker, *Haunted Memories*, 10.
31. Sealey, "Camp Creek Wreck."
32. *Atlanta Constitution*, "Fast Train," 5.

Chapter Four

33. *Jackson-Argus*, "Awful Wreck."
34. Ibid.
35. Ibid.
36. Ibid.
37. *Henry County Weekly*, "Horror of Horrors."
38. *Macon Telegraph*, "Thirty-Three Lives Lost," 1.

Chapter Five

39. Ibid.
40. *Henry County Weekly*, "Horror of Horrors."
41. Ibid.
42. Ibid.; and *Macon Telegraph*, "Thirty Three Lives Lost."
43. *Macon Telegraph*, "Thirty Three Lives Lost."
44. Ibid.

45. *Henry County Weekly*, "Horror of Horrors."
46. *Macon Telegraph*, "Thirty Three Lives Lost."
47. Ibid.
48. Ibid.
49. Ibid.
50. Ibid.; and Carey, "Dead Number Thirty Three," 6.
51. *Macon Telegraph*, "Thirty Three Lives Lost."
52. Carey, "Thirty One Lives Lost," 1.
53. Carey, "Dead Number Thirty Three," 6.
54. *Henry County Weekly*, "Horror of Horrors."
55. Ibid.
56. *Macon Telegraph*, "Thirty Three Lives Lost."
57. *Macon Telegraph*, "Hunting Bodies."
58. *Macon Telegraph*, "Thirty Three Lives Lost."
59. Ibid.

CHAPTER SIX

60. Ibid.
61. Carey, "Dead Number Thirty Three," 6.
62. Carey, "Thirty One Lives Lost," 1.
63. *Macon Telegraph*, "No More Bodies," 1.
64. Ibid.
65. Ibid.
66. *Macon Telegraph*, "Hunting Bodies."
67. Ibid.
68. Rainer, *Henry County, Georgia*, 329.
69. *Atlanta Constitution*, "He Was Buried as an Unknown," 7.
70. *Atlanta Constitution*, "Bodies of Wreck Victims," 2.
71. Ibid.
72. *Atlanta Constitution*, "Funeral of Captain Barclay," 4.
73. *Macon Telegraph*, "Thirty Three Lives Lost," 2.
74. *Atlanta Constitution*, "Thomas J. Malone," 6.
75. Reed, J.T. Sullivan's Grave.
76. *Atlanta Constitution*, "Funeral Notices," 10.
77. Sealey, "Camp Creek Wreck."
78. *Atlanta Constitution*, "Twelve Atlantans," 5. See also "About Us."
79. Ibid.

80. Ibid.
81. *Macon Telegraph*, "Hunting Bodies," 5.
82. Ibid.
83. Ibid.
84. Rainer, *Henry County, Georgia*, 329.
85. Ibid.
86. *Atlanta Constitution*, "Wreck Victim Identified," 4.
87. Ibid.
88. *Atlanta Constitution*, "One More Body Recovered," 5.
89. *Macon Telegraph*, "Hunting Bodies."
90. Ibid.

Chapter Seven

91. *Atlanta Constitution*, "Locomotive 846," 5.
92. Ibid.
93. *Macon Telegraph*, "Hunting Bodies."
94. *Atlanta Constitution*, "Inevitable Act of God," 5.
95. Ibid.
96. *Atlanta Constitution*, "Prompt Payment," 5.
97. *Atlanta Constitution*, "Act of God," 12. See also *Atlanta Constitution*, "Camp Creek Cases," 12.
98. Maysilles, "Hoke Smith."
99. *Atlanta Constitution*, "Act of God."
100. Rainer, *Henry County, Georgia*, 329.
101. *Atlanta Constitution*, "His Life Worth," 12.
102. *Atlanta Constitution*, "No New Developments," 5.
103. *Atlanta Constitution*, "Bob Spencer's Four Widows," 2.

Selected Bibliography

Newspaper Articles

Atlanta Constitution. "Are No New Developments." May 11, 1901.

———. "Bad Washout Near Luella." June 25, 1900.

———. "Bob Spencer's Four Widows." March 29, 1901.

———. "Bodies of Wreck Victims Arrive." June 25, 1900.

———. "Camp Creek Cases Come Up in April." March 26, 1901.

———. "Defendant Pleads an Act of God." February 7, 1901.

———. "Fast Train Drops into a Ditch Near Atlanta." June 24, 1900.

———. "Funeral Notices: Sullivan." June 25, 1900.

———. "Funeral of Captain Barclay: He Was Laid to Rest in Selma, Ala." June 29, 1900.

———. "He Was Buried as an Unknown." July 12, 1900.

————. "His Life Worth $100,000." July 12, 1900.

————. "Locomotive 846 Has Bloody Record." June 25, 1900.

————. "One More Body Is Recovered." June 27, 1900.

————. "Prompt Payment." July 25, 1900.

————. "Southern Officials Say Wreck Is an Inevitable Act of God." June 25, 1900.

————. "Thomas J. Malone Died Yesterday." December 27, 1901.

————. "Twelve Atlantans Were Victims of the Disaster on Southern at M'Donough Saturday Night." June 25, 1900.

————. "Wreck Victim Is Identified." June 29, 1900.

Carey, Daniel. "Dead Number Thirty Three; Six Bodies Are Identified." *Atlanta Constitution*, June 26, 1900.

————. "Thirty One Lives Lost in M'Donough Disaster; Greatest Loss of Life Known in Southern Wreck." *Atlanta Constitution*, June 25, 1900.

Henry County Weekly. "Horror of Horrors: Wild Plunge of a Passenger Train into Camp Creek Culvert." June 29, 1900, vol. XXV.

Jackson-Argus. "Awful Wreck: Many Lives Lost in Camp Creek Disaster." June 29, 1900.

Macon Telegraph. "Hunting Bodies From the Wreck." June 26, 1900.
————. "No More Bodies Will Be Found." June 27, 1900.

————. "Thirty Three Lives Lost in Wreck on Southern." June 25, 1900.

New York Times. "Samuel Spencer Killed in Wreck." November 30, 1906.

Sealey, C.L. "Buddy." "Camp Creek Wreck Remembered." *Henry Daily Herald*, June 21, 2000.

BOOKS

Bailey, Anne J. *The Chessboard of War: Sherman and Hood in the Autumn Campaigns of 1864*. Lincoln: University of Nebraska Press, 2000.

Bowen, Rhoda Anne, and Fred R. Turner, eds. *Georgia Confederate Soldiers Obituaries: Henry, Newton and Rockdale Counties: 1879–1943*. Alpharetta, GA: W.H. Wolfe Associates Historical Publications, 1992.

Brooks, Dan, and Caprice Walker. *Haunted Memories of McDonough, Georgia*. McDonough, GA: Privately Published, 2006.

Cook, James F. *Governors of Georgia: 1754–1995*. Macon, GA: Mercer University Press, 1995.

Coulter, E. Merton. *Georgia: A Short History*. Chapel Hill: University of North Carolina Press, 1933.

Morris, Gene, Jr. *True Southerners: A Pictorial History of Henry County, Georgia*. McDonough, GA: Henry County Records Publishers, 2000.

Rainer, Vessie Thrasher. *Henry County, Georgia: The Mother of Counties*. McDonough, GA: Privately Published, 1971.

Speer, Scip. *History of Henry County: 1821–1921*. Hampton, GA: Rocky Creek Social Club, 1988.

Sullivan, Buddy, and the Georgia Historical Society. *Georgia: A State History*. Charleston, SC: Arcadia Publishing, 2003.

Trudeau, Noah Andre. *Southern Storm: Sherman's March to the Sea*. New York: Harper Collins, 2008.

Wells, Jeffery. *Moments in McDonough History*. McDonough, GA: Privately Published, 2009.

WEB ARTICLES

"About Us." *Haverty's*. www.havertys.com, accessed August 1, 2009.

"East Tennessee, Virginia & Georgia Railroad." *Railga.com.* http://railga.com/etvg.html, accessed July 29, 2009.

"Macon & Brunswick Railroad." *RailGa.com.* http://railga.com/macbrun.html, accessed July 29, 2009.

Maysilles, Duncan. "Hoke Smith (1855–1931)." *New Georgia Encyclopedia.* www.newgeorgiaencyclopedia.com, accessed December 19, 2008.

"Samuel Spencer." *Railway and Locomotive Historical Society.* http://rlhs.org/rlhsnews/htms/nl26-4.htm#spencer, accessed February 18, 2009.

"Southern Railway History." *Southern Railway Historical Association.* http://www.srha.net/public/History/history.htm, accessed February 18, 2009.

E-MAIL

Reed, Sam. J.T. Sullivan's Grave at Oakland. E-mail to author, January 26, 2009.

About the Author

Jeffery Wells is assistant professor of history and department chair at Georgia Military College's Atlanta campus. In addition to writing for his popular blog, "Georgia Mysteries," Wells is working on a book about Georgia's Bigfoot (forthcoming from Idyl Arbor Press). He has written articles for the New Georgia Encyclopedia online and chapters for the Georgia Criterion Reference Test on Georgia History. He is a member of the Georgia Association of Historians, the Southern Historical Association, Clayton/Henry County Genealogical Society and the Robert Penn Warren Circle. He serves as guest presenter for McDonough Haunted History Tours in conjunction with local bookstore Bell, Book & Candle. He has a short article on the Camp Creek Crash forthcoming in *Georgia Backroads* magazine (Fall 2009).

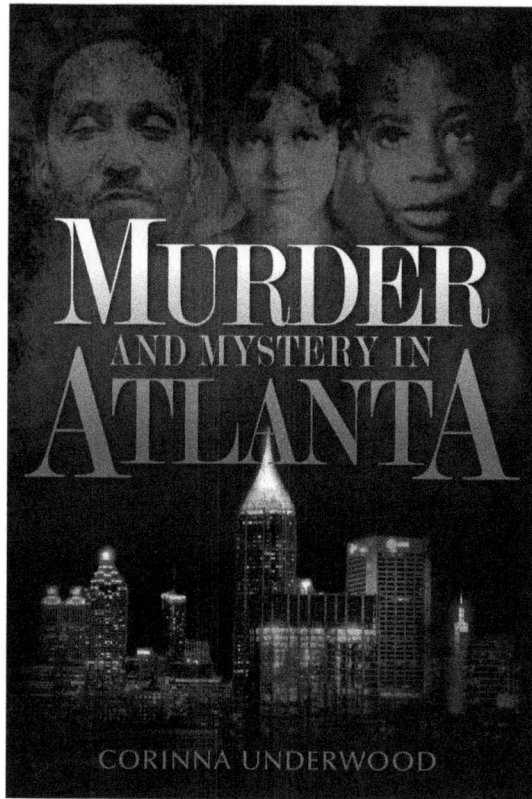

CORINNA UNDERWOOD

If you enjoyed this book, you may also enjoy Corrina Underwood's
Murder and Mystery in Atlanta

$19.99 • 128 pages • 30 images • ISBN 978-1-59629-766-1

Atlanta, the largest city in the Southeast, hides a dark and violent past. Join local author Corinna Underwood as she investigates some of Atlanta's most notorious crimes, many of which are unsolved, from the city's first homicide to its gender hate crimes. Who really killed young Mary Phagan in an Atlanta pencil factory? Was there really an Atlanta Ripper, or was it just a series of copycat killings? After reading these chilling accounts, you'll be sure to lock your door.

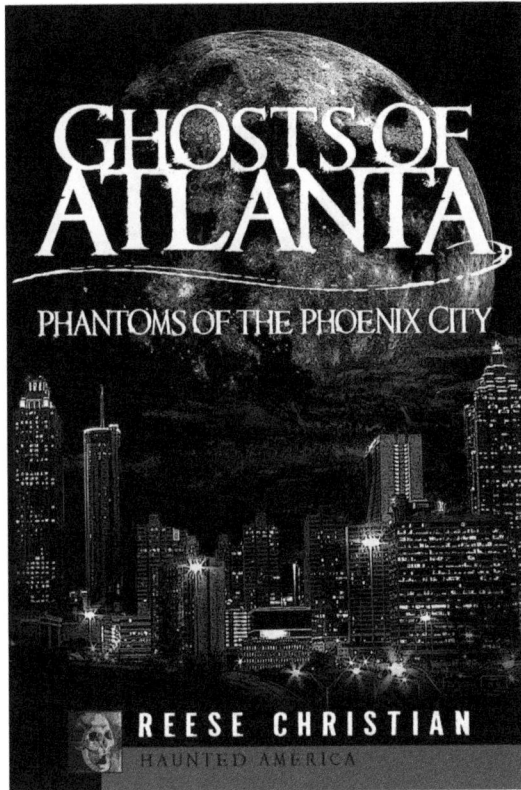

If you enjoyed this book, you may also enjoy Reese Christian's
Ghosts of Atlanta: Phantoms of the Phoenix City

$19.99 • 128 pages • Over 70 images • ISBN 978-1-59629-544-5

Drawing on her work with the Cold Case Investigative Research Institute at Bauder College and Ghost Hounds Paranormal Research Society, elite psychic medium and cold case researcher Reese Christian writes of the tragic past and the haunted present of Greater Atlanta. From Peachtree Street in the heart of downtown to the plantations and battlefields surrounding the city, join her in discovering the twisted histories of some of Atlanta's most infamous landmarks and forgotten moments.

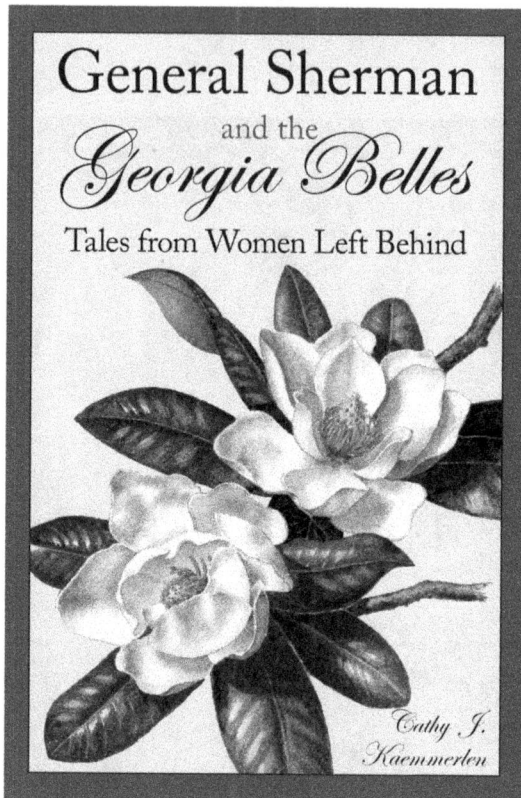

General Sherman
and the
Georgia Belles
Tales from Women Left Behind

Cathy J.
Kaemmerlen

If you enjoyed this book, you may also enjoy Cathy J. Kaemmerlen's
General Sherman and the Georgia Belles:
Tales from Women Left Behind

$19.99 • 128 pages • Over 11 images • ISBN 978-1-59629-159-1

As Sherman and his troops marched to the sea, Georgians, particularly brave women looking to defend their families, scrambled to protect their homes from this infamous campaign—using not only their Southern belle charm, but their ingenuity as well. In every sense "steel magnolias," Georgia's women stood on their front porches and bravely faced sixty thousand invading Federal soldiers.

Despite the devastation and fear Sherman and his troops inflicted, the Georgia belles were poised to stand firm in the face of an invasion and, as Martha Amanda Quillin phrases it, "We contended for every principle of honor and justice and for the most sacred rights—FOR THE SANCTITY OF HOME."

Cathy Kaemmerlen, a renowned storyteller and historical interpreter, provides a colorful collection of tales of exceptional Georgia women who made great sacrifices in an effort to save their familics and homes. From the innocent diary of a ten-year-old girl to the words of a woman who risks everything to see her husband one last time, Kaemmerlen exposes the grit and gumption of these remarkable Southern women in an inspiring and entertaining fashion.

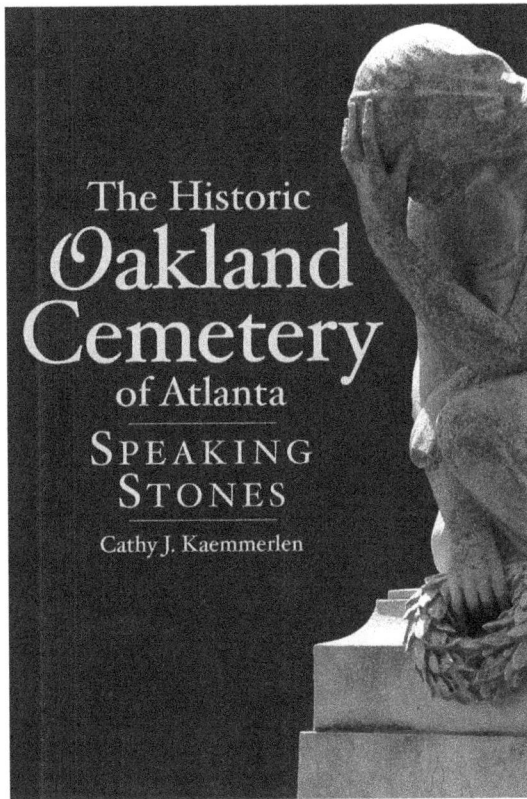

Visit us at
www.historypress.net